Endorsements

Every thirty seconds, a woman is diagnosed with breast cancer. In the United States, comprehensive screening programs and state-of-the art treatments have achieved survival rates of over eighty percent. In other countries, including India, survival continues to be less than thirty percent, primarily driven by advanced stages at presentation.

With the rising incidence of breast cancer in India, a new voice is needed, not only to increase awareness but also to provide hope for those who find themselves on this lonely, unfamiliar road. I am privileged to know Aley. Her story is real and provides insight into a life-changing event. A potentially deadly mass of cells brought out a strength and courage that I suspect she did not even know she had. Aley's understanding of the Bible and its practical, daily application to her new world of medical interventions and interactions will certainly be an inspiration to people of any religion.

Aley's book will serve as a bridge for patients, families, and friends, traversing the difficult waters between the lands of cancer and survival.

Roshni Rao MD, FACS
Assistant Professor
Dept. of Surgery, Division of Surgical Oncology
Vice Chief of Staff, UTSW Zale Hospital

The book entitled *Blessings of My Breast Cancer* by Aley Abraham is a profoundly fascinating and inspiring work. It is a sublime response and articulation of a noble Christian who encounters the most shocking experience of fatal cancer disease. The Author's internal dialectical conflicts are vivid, and the search for the meaning of a brutal malignancy are found in the writings. A radical transition from an experience of shock and frustration to an unconditional faith submission, acceptance, meaning, hope and tranquility in life is beautifully unveiled in the book. This book could be recommended as a spiritual reading and therapy text for cancer patients and inspirational literature for all those who are in pursuit of peace and meaning in life. I am sure the book will have extensive readership, and wish the Author Aley Abraham God's choicest blessings.

Dr. Philipos Mar Stephanos
Auxiliary Bishop
Archdiocese of Tiruvalla, India

I am happy to recommend the Book, *Blessings of My Breast Cancer*, by Aley Abraham. The authenticity of the book lies in personal experience of going through the dreaded sickness of cancer. To hear about the disease and to go through the sickness are not the same. The reader will get a blend of these two experiences through the chapters of this book. The traumatic experience of recognizing that one is a cancer patient can turn the life for good or bad. In Aley Abraham, the reader will find a transformed person with deeper faith, entering into theological reflections and learning greater Biblical truths. Therefore, the book is a scholarly work, full of life's experiences, medical treatments, biblical truths, and theological insights.

I congratulate Aley Abraham for the good work. I wish and pray that this book illuminates the lives of innumerable people to recognize that life is [they are] "fearfully and wonderfully made" by God.

Geevarghese Mar Theodosius, Ph.D.
Bishop - Mar Thoma Church
Diocese of North America & Europe

Blessings of My Breast Cancer

Written by Aley Abraham

with Susan Abraham Thomas

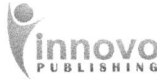

innovo
PUBLISHING

Published by
Innovo Publishing, LLC
www.innovopublishing.com
1-888-546-2111

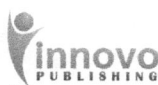

innovo
PUBLISHING

Providing Full-Service Publishing Services for
Christian Authors, Artists & Organizations: Hardbacks, Paperbacks,
eBooks, Audiobooks, Music & Videos

Unless otherwise indicated, Scripture is taken from Bible Gateway,
New International Version, www.biblegateway.com.
Bible Gateway, American Standard Version, www.biblegateway.com.
Bible Gateway, New American Standard Bible, www.biblegateway.com.

Library of Congress Control Number: 2012950094
ISBN 13: 978-1-61314-060-4

Cover Design & Interior Layout: Innovo Publishing, LLC

Printed in the United States of America
U.S. Printing History

First Edition: October 2012

Dedicated to my late beloved father, P. M. Varghese,
who loved me very much, and my late beloved mother,
Sosamma Varghese, a simple, humble, and very godly woman
who taught me through her life that "Blessed are those who have
regard for the weak; the LORD delivers them
in times of trouble" (Psalm 41:1).
I admire her the most.

Mom, I wanted to give you a copy of the book. Sorry I was not
able to. I am very grateful for your example.
I love you so much.

To both, thank you so much for being great parents.

Acknowledgments

First and foremost, I thank my God who has solidified my faith through the sickness of cancer; who has healed both my body and my spirit; who has removed feelings of hopelessness, fear, and anxiety; who has provided hope, courage, and self-confidence; who has given me a steadfast mind; and who has chosen me as a vehicle to write this book, just as Jesus chose the donkey as a vehicle to ride.

Writing and publishing this book has been the biggest accomplishment of my life but without the support and compassion of my family and friends, none of this would have been realized. So I want to thank the following people.

Susan Abraham Thomas, my beloved daughter who put all my thoughts into words. Because of your passion for Christ, you made time for me and were diligent for me. Without your dedication, this project would not have been possible. I want to extend my personal sincere thanks to you.

Benji Philips, my second daughter, and her friend, Smitha Jones, for helping me to edit this book.

My son-in-law, Dr. Binu Philips, for helping to edit the chapter about medical terminology and for the research you provided in finding a good doctor.

My son-in-law, B. J. Thomas, for your love for God and helping me with support groups.

My precious jewel and my grandbaby, Abriana, for your innocent prayers.

The strong prayer warriors (Lizey, Lilly, Valsa, Lizy, and Mary) who came to my house and prayed for me with such conviction.

Estella for always giving me a shoulder to cry on and for providing hope in the midst of my dark times.

To my immediate family: Mathew and family, Mammen and family, Ann and family, Varghese and family for supporting me. Alex and family, and Philip and family—you all loved me the most and supported me. I love you all so much.

My surgeon, Dr. Roshni Rao, and my oncologist, Dr. Jenny Li, for their love for patients and their dedication to their trade.

American Cancer Society through whom I got help from the volunteers of the University of the Southwestern Medical Center.

I thank God for Innovo Publishing, who was able to supply encouragement in such a way that built up my confidence. I never saw them as a business entity, but as a caring entity that understood the needs of a new author. Every word supplied by them was filled with grace. A special thanks to my editor, Darya Crockett, who guided me patiently through the process and understood the limitations I had in this new endeavor.

And most of all my beloved husband, Abraham Kulathumkal, for your unconditional love for the past thirty-nine years. You were a teacher of the Bible, a nurse for all of my wounds, a husband in every way, and a counselor for all of my needs. When God gave me a husband, He gave me the best. I love you.

Foreword

The pages in this book reflect a deep, spiritual journey, which began in Aley's life following her diagnosis of breast cancer. Aley displays a remarkably honest presentation of her feelings, initially of great despair, and then of hope, based on her relationship with God and the promises that He has made through the generations to surround us "with the songs of deliverance." The book takes the reader on a journey on earth in which Aley struggles with the diagnosis, walks through a mastectomy and chemotherapy, comes to understand her greater purpose in life. Then the cycle begins again as her brother is diagnosed with breast cancer and Aley learns that she carries the gene that increases the likelihood of having recurrent cancer and increases the possibility that her daughters will have cancer as well. The partnership with God that she has developed throughout the journey, with a constant intertwining of early experience with spirituality and scripture, reflects the final outcome of her story, where she shares that "Cancer was my spiritual training ground. It transformed my mind." And so, Aley considers the trials she has seen to be a blessing, which has allowed her to achieve a closer relationship with God and to share the wisdom and peace she has grown to embody.

On a personal note, I had the wonderful opportunity to work with, and learn from, Aley. She is someone who walked through her trials with courage, although it is clear from the text of this book that her outward courage was visible even though there was great inner conflict. As difficult as life was for her during this time, she was a constant source of support for all those around her, including me, when we needed a word of encouragement. She is a testament to her faith, and her journey has indeed produced great strength in a way that she would not have anticipated.

One phrase that is reflected throughout her text is a verse from Philippians, which is bundled into four daily reflections of victory over despair. These tenets read:

1. Nothing is impossible for God.
2. I can do everything through Him who gives me strength.
3. God chose me, even as a cancer patient. Just as he searched for the donkey on which the Son of God should ride, God chose me to be a vessel to fill.
4. I am a victor. God's favor is upon me. Even though I am weak, I become strong through Him.

The journey to the depths of despair, regardless of what has sent a person to that lonely place, provides a rich ground on which God plants the seeds of strength—strength made from a true partnership between God and those of us who He loves so dearly. The trials of life are a gift from which growth and understanding arise, so that we may better share the wisdom we gain when we travel to the loneliest of places. God rescued Aley from that lonely place, and the shining, bright woman that emerged has shared her story so that others who travel this journey may find hope, strength, and peace.

Beverly B. Rogers, MD
Chief of Pathology, Children's Healthcare of Atlanta
Adjunct Professor of Pathology, Emory University School of Medicine

Aley and I were colleagues in the laboratory at Children's Medical Center Dallas for over six years. We did not have a close relationship, at least, not in the traditional sense, but it always felt like we were close somehow. While our conversations were not lengthy, they were always memorable.

Our conversations were never about the weather, the local sports teams, or other topics, which are the stuff of short, casual exchanges. No, our conversations were about life's purpose, the elements of our existence that provide meaning. In that vein, we talked about theology, about our families, and about leaders like Mahatma Gandhi and Abraham Lincoln, who we felt were great because of their spiritual substance and because they led in order to serve.

In looking back, I realize our close connection may have been related to two things. First, as the lab's senior director, I wrote an article in our monthly department newsletter. I usually wrote about different aspects of the same theme—encouraging staff to view their time working as more than just earning a paycheck, but as a sacred calling that offers purpose, worthwhile work, and the opportunity to make a positive difference in the lives of others. Second, because Aley actually read the articles and seriously considered what they meant for her. Perhaps that was why our conversations started so easily with substantive topics, and that may explain her kind invitation to write this foreword.

Aley would often approach me with a comment about a recent article I had written, and we easily fell into conversation on topics of significance and relevance, such as challenging the mental models and biases with which we viewed the world and others. Or we would re-create the myths about who we are, myths that had been given to us as youths by our teachers and parents, and encouraged behaviors and a self-identity that worked against our happiness and purpose.

What we had in common was the belief that our work actually was a sacred calling and that each day was part of our spiritual journeys. This was what we talked about on the commuter train, during the walks from the train to the hospital, or during breaks at work.

Aley offers you a similar conversation in this book. It is personal. It is emotional. It is about self, family, and relationships. It is about sickness and healing. It is about anxiety, dread, worry, death, happiness, joy, and profound fulfillment. It vacillates between life's ecstatic highs and devastating lows. It is substantive. It is a powerful story, beautifully written.

The essential message focuses on Aley's maturing relationship with God and herself. Starting with God as protector who helps her conquer her fears—the God described in the 23rd Psalm—the journey ends with God as personal co-creator of life and meaning.

Aley's struggle with breast cancer is a metaphor for humankind's struggle with meaninglessness, emptiness, and fear. Her story is about the realization that without a personal God, the struggle will not be a joyful one. Through her story, Aley teaches us that to struggle is to be alive, and the struggle will be a profoundly joyful one if we let it. It depends on the choices we make. We are in control. We can relate to God as a concept to satisfy our aesthetic feelings and intellectual needs, or we can relate to God as a Being who is personal and with whom we co-create our lives in the best possible way. As the philosopher Schelling said, "Only a person can heal a person."

It is the person-to-Person relationship, or being-to-Being relationship, or as Martin Buber called it, the I-Thou relationship, that Aley discovered through her struggle with breast cancer, and that is why she came to view her breast cancer as a gift. Aley chose the gift over the curse, and that made all the difference. Her choice allowed community with her personal God and brought her strength, joy, and healing. The truth she discovered is that the healing will always be with Aley, whether or not the sickness stays away.

Aley's goal is to share her experience to help others. Every one of us has our own challenge that represents either a dreaded curse we must endure or a gift by which we can achieve the true understanding of what is possible. Aley knows we all must make that choice. She writes, "My hope is that others can learn from my mistakes and alter their future by it." That statement invites you into the pages beyond.

James L. Adams
Administrative Director, Laboratory
Children's Healthcare of Atlanta

Contents

Prologue

*M*y beloved father passed away from a terminal disease called cancer, specifically prostate gland cancer. Seeing his suffering, pain, and hopelessness broke my heart. The sickness was so devastating and brought such great fear to my life that I wished deeply that even my worst enemy would never have to endure the pain of cancer. I began to develop a deep compassion for cancer patients and wanted to offer help in some way. Financially, my father's treatment and care was expensive, so I thought that maybe I could offer monetary help to cancer patients who could not afford it themselves. But to this day, I have not been able to offer that support. Little did I know that finances were just a small part of cancer's toll. Twenty-one years later, I myself became a cancer patient. It came as a shock and my mind began to focus on the dreadful call of death. I was filled with fear of death, guilt, hopelessness, and a feeling of isolation. I thought it was the end of my life All of a sudden, I realized how simple my thinking was during my father's time of sickness, as the only way I could fathom helping other cancer patients was to provide for them financially. But dealing with the emotions of cancer was harder than the physical pain of the mastectomy and the complications of the chemotherapy's side effects. I realized the need to be freed from all of my negative feelings. During my time of crisis, I began to meditate like I had never done before. My meditations led me to accept this as MY SICKNESS. It was painful both physically and emotionally, but I had to endure. Neither the doctors nor my family and friends could take my pain for me. Only God could deliver me. When I understood this truth, I drew close to God, and God gave me the wonderful gift of deliverance—deliverance of my past sins. He gave me thoughts of jubilee. I received strength from above.

Now, I want to pass on this truth. I want to express my deliverance in writing so that others can also benefit. Although I once desired to help cancer patients in a limited way through finances, I hope that this book will bring both financial as well as emotional support. Perhaps that is why God had allowed me to endure cancer— to receive an empathetic heart.

As a breast cancer survivor, I believe that healing involves the mind, body, and spirit. Today, I believe that my cancer was not my end. Rather, it was just the beginning of a new life that would be used to encourage and inspire others who have lost hope. What a blessing!

Proceeds from this book will be distributed to the unfortunate cancer patients who cannot afford treatment themselves and to the education of children who have lost their parent(s) to cancer.

Aley Abraham

What I feared has come upon me; what I dreaded has happened to me. (Job 3:25)

In 1986, my beloved father was diagnosed with prostate gland cancer and the doctor said he only had six months left to live. My family in India informed me of this terrible news and I immediately booked a flight to travel thousands of miles from Dallas, Texas, to the Madras Cancer Institute in Madras, India, where my father was being treated. I went straight from the airport to the hospital and saw a man that I hardly recognized. Growing up, my father was a very strong, capable man who held a reputable position in the society, but in that hospital bed I saw a man who had lost an incredible amount of weight, who looked feeble and completely incapable of holding even a glass of water on his own. Although I had never seen my father cry, his eyes were brimming with tears in that hospital bed. His disposition evoked alarming shock within my soul.

Although the doctors had informed our family that he only had six months left to live, it was not customary to tell the patient himself. I asked my father what the doctors had told him, and he stated that he would be fine if he just went back home. I was too afraid to state the matter to him as well, because I knew the gravity of the situation and knew that he was getting closer to death with each day. He was never a complainer, so he never expressed the pain he was in, but I could see from the expressions on his face and from the straining he went through that he was in such incredible pain, and it broke my heart. The sickness was so devastating that the deepest part of my heart hoped that this type of suffering would never come upon even my worst enemy. What I experienced kindled dread toward the disease, and it awoke within me *sensitivity* to the needs of cancer patients. At that moment, I knew that I wanted to financially help cancer patients who could not afford treatment themselves.

That following Christmas, nine months after he was diagnosed, my father passed away. Twenty-one years later, in June 2007, I was diagnosed with breast cancer, and I realized that finances were just a small part of a much larger problem. While I was financially secure, emotionally I was not.

I couldn't believe it. The diagnosis came at the most unexpected time. I had just come back from a month-long vacation; my youngest daughter had just graduated from law school. It was a happy time in my life. I went in for a routine mammogram, and I got a call at work from the hospital asking me to come in and repeat the test.

"Why?" I asked.

They said they found some calcification on a mass in the breast and wanted to test again. At that moment, a thought entered my head that I may have cancer, but not wanting to hear such a diagnosis, I dismissed the thought. But after the second test, a biopsy result confirmed that I had invasive ductal carcinoma, otherwise known as cancer.

INVASIVE DUCTAL CARCINOMA. Oh my goodness. What was happening? I couldn't comprehend everything that was being said. I did not want to hear it. Fear immediately took over. How could the one thing that I feared the most be happening to me? I knew cancer was a deadly disease and that my days were numbered. I could not sleep, I could not eat, and I lost all of my strength. Fear had control. Fear overpowered me. Fear took the place of emotional stability and reasoning. I could not focus on anything. I had lost all hope. I could not enjoy life. I had died inside.

I called my boss at work and informed her that I would not be able to come back to work at all. I thought I was dying and felt that I could not go back to work. So I sat at home for a few days by myself focusing on my disease. I was afraid to look at my breast. My eldest daughter and her husband tried consoling me by bringing me to their home to pass time. They spoke words of encouragement and put on religious TV programs to help me overcome my fear, but none of that helped. I was not in a state of mind to receive anything positive. Although I grew up reading the Bible, I could not remember one word of hope from it. I was drowning in fear. And I was restless. I could not be consoled by any human being.

As a cancer patient, I felt isolated from my society, and I felt that the community saw my days as being numbered. My husband would try to get me to go to church, and I would resist because I did not want to feel the weight of my community's sympathies toward me. I believed that they saw cancer as the most deadly disease to ever come upon man, and I was afraid to face their fears.

One Sunday, when my husband somehow convinced me to attend church, I saw some members crying in the hallway. I immediately thought they were crying because of my ill circumstances and this brought great fear upon me. I felt that they were looking at me as a lamb brought to its slaughter. I FELT DEATH and it afflicted me. Then I came to find out that the mourners were saddened over the death of our priest's father, who had passed away from cancer. This news came as both a relief and as an added weight. To top it off, I was also reminded of another church member who was battling a severe form of cancer. Cancer seemed to be all around me and my fears mounted.

Many cancer patients received healing, complete healing. I grew up seeing my neighbor survive forty long years after her battle with breast cancer. However, rather than see the positive of her experience, my mind kept recalling the more negative experience of my father's quick demise nine months after he was diagnosed with cancer. I was plagued with the fear of death, and I was not ready for the Creator's judgment of me.

I looked in my closet filled with beautiful saris and felt despair that I would no longer be able to wear any of them because I would die soon. I had suddenly lost my interest in clothes and jewelry—I lost my interest in life. I wished my doctor had never told me this devastating news.

I woke up Monday morning to an empty house and a mind filled with the same fear from the days past. I was suffocating.

I needed some relief. I did not have anyone to console me. Out of desperation, I cried unto God. I begged Him to show me something, anything. I remembered the story of Job and his sufferings, and I opened up my Bible to read about him. I arrived at Job 5:18–20:

For he wounds, but he also binds up; he injures, but his hands also heal. From six calamities he will rescue you; in seven no harm will touch you. In famine he will deliver you from death, and in battle from the stroke of the sword.

This verse brought me some hope. I felt as if God was right beside me assuring me that I would not die until my appointed time. I felt that I would live well into my aging days. I remembered my neighbor's healing from breast cancer and I began to hope.

My prayer is that no one person would have to endure such trials in her mind. God Himself came and wrapped me up in His arms, and He alone was my comforter.

Cancer of the body can be removed and treated with chemotherapy and surgery, but the cancer in the mind is not treatable by worldly doctors. Only the Word of God can destroy the cancer in your mind. My hope is that this book will communicate how God freed me from my captivity and strengthened me to take more responsibility than I ever had in my life. I hope that you can benefit from my experiences during your times of trial.

Fear assaults insight and reason. In unexpected times of trouble, we develop a fear of death because we live life void of thoughts of our last days. So we must think often about death while we are living. We should also think often about the judgment of God. No one will live forever; all must face death and then judgment. If we think of the end of life and judgment often, it will lead us to belief in Christ, belief in God, and it will convince us to seek salvation. It will lead us to read and meditate on the Word of God, which will weave courage, fortitude, and endurance within. Then when trouble knocks on our door, we will not suddenly be struck with panic. Instead, we will realize that sickness is just another part of life, and this perception will help us to live life to the fullest, even in the midst of suffering.

What a wretched man I am! Who will rescue
me from this body that is subject to death?
(Romans 7:24)

Paul, a well-known figure in the Bible and one of the greatest apostles of Christ, used to be known as Saul before his great conversion. Saul was strong in his religious views as a Jew persecuting the Christian Church. The Bible says he was a Pharisee of the Pharisees, meaning he was like the Arch Bishop. He was strict in his views and headstrong. It was during one of his persecutions that the Lord visited him in a sea of light, blinding his sight, and it was through the loss of his worldly views that he was able to gain insight into the person of Jehovah God. It was this zealot, in the middle of his personal ambitions, whom God chose to alter.

What a conversion it was! He who once persecuted the church was now being persecuted. He who once was zealous for the written law was now zealous for the love of Christ. Paul was a changed man in his thoughts and actions, and he lived only for Christ. He was able to perform great miracles and people saw him as a god. But even this man, dedicated as he was, cried out, "Oh wretched man that I am! Who will deliver me from this body of death?"

He *groaned.*

This theologian. This man who was caught up in the third heaven. This super-Christian.

He was frustrated. He was agitated because he could not rid himself of the evil inside. Though he was saved and had experienced

21

wondrous things of the Lord and had solid faith, he still struggled with the ungodliness of his ways. He couldn't do what he wanted to do.

In the same way that Paul could not rid himself of his sins, I also struggled with my flesh. Even though I had received some hope that I would not die, at times I would lose hope. Fear and guilt would enter along with hopelessness and sadness. God had promised me life, but I could not take hold of it. The fear of death was so much greater than the hope that God offered. Death was like a python slithering after me with large jaws open wide. I could not escape the fear.

When my doctor suggested chemotherapy and a mastectomy, my family took all sorts of initiatives to ensure that I was being given the best treatment possible. My son-in-law, who was a doctor himself, heavily researched the surgeon and the center. My daughters sent emails to the surgeon to ask a myriad of questions. My older son-in-law poured over the Internet to find as much information as he could, and my husband asked all sorts of questions to my doctor. But even though all efforts were taken to secure the best treatment possible, I remained void of hope. I remember going into my closet to let my tears flow in secret because I did not want my family to also lose hope by seeing me in my state of despair. At that moment, I longed deeply for someone to come with a word of hope, a word of encouragement. But it seemed that no one was able to give that to me. Some who came approached me with sadness in their hearts and tears in their eyes. They themselves had no hope, so they could not give hope. Their despondent spirit brought my spirit down even lower. Others, although they had a word of encouragement, I could not receive it because I was so downcast.

I understood through this trial that one of the most difficult jobs in the world was to "encourage the disheartened" (1 Thessalonians 5:14). I understood that only those who received the Holy Spirit would be able to give this type of comfort because they have no fear of death. Those who have the Holy Spirit possess hope—*I wanted that*. I did not want to be afraid of death any longer. I wanted to have hope and to give hope to others who may be going through similar trials. I wanted to be freed from my bondage of fear, and I cried out to God for my release.

I wished greatly that just one person could offer some comfort and could tell me that everything was going to be all right. I realized that it was an extremely difficult task. I also had a desire to offer this comfort to other sufferers.

I was a slave of disbelief. Rather than believing that my sins were forgiven freely, I remained in the control of disbelief. In the same way that Paul cried out to God, I also cried out to God in brokenness, begging Him to give me some relief. I could not handle the pain of anxiety and fear. No one could save me. Salvation could come only from God. My soul was crying out for salvation. Then, God in His mercy poured out His grace and gave me a word:

[David said] "Then I acknowledged my sin to you and did not cover up my iniquity. I said, 'I will confess my transgressions to the Lord.' And you forgave the guilt of my sin. Therefore let all the faithful pray to you while you may be found; surely the rising of the mighty waters will not reach them. You are my hiding place; you will protect me from trouble and surround me with songs of deliverance." [God said] "I will instruct you and teach you in the way you should go; I will counsel you with my loving eye on you" (Psalm 32:5–8).

These verses convicted me and urged me to confess my sins to the Lord. In a way, I was longing for forgiveness. I began to understand that the real reason for my restlessness and anxiety was caused by sin inhabiting my mind; in other words, I was a slave of unbelief and sin. God promised me an eternity in heaven but considering my disregard for the Word of God, I felt I was unworthy of His forgiveness. I believed that I had too many transgressions and that I could not accept these promises from God. The realization of my lack of faith prompted me to imitate David, the king, to go to the Lord with a humble and believing heart of a child. As I started my confession and repentance, it gave me hope that I was not too far from the kingdom of God and that I too could attain salvation. The confirmation of such a hope instilled and grew in me day by day, which gave me the realization that I was on my way to eternity in heaven, and God's promise was becoming real in my life.

My lack of belief was the biggest sin. I thought I believed, but in reality when my faith was tested, I recognized that I did not have enough conviction. I repented for my lack of faith and asked God for forgiveness. I needed Him and asked Him to help me trust His promises. So when I finally found the courage to pray during my cancer, I did not ask for physical healing; I asked for healing for my soul. And God, in His great mercy, provided both.

I began my prayers with the words that David used when he asked God for forgiveness: *"Create in me a clean heart, O God and renew a steadfast spirit within me" (Psalm 51:10).*

I began to trust his promise that He would give good gifts to those who asked: *"Or if he asks for a fish, will give him a snake? If you, then, though you are evil, know how to give good gifts to your children, how much more will your Father in heaven give good gifts to those who ask him!" (Matthew 7:10–11).*

I saw my heavenly Father as an even greater parental figure than my own loving earthly father. Out of six siblings, I was my father's favorite. He spoiled me and gave me anything I asked for. That was his love for me. I am also a mother. My happiness lies in my children's well-being. Giving them what they desire brings me joy. But my earthly father was taken away from me, and I will also be taken away from my children. What you receive from your earthly parents is limited. But our heavenly Father, who is the Creator of this universe, is able to give more than we can even imagine. He alone can forgive sins, and He is surpassingly loving and forgiving, so we do not have to worry about anything. When I had this epiphany, I knew that no matter what I asked for, He could provide. Whether it was empathizing with my feelings or removing my sadness and fears, my God was sufficient. You can believe what the Word of God says. It is the Word of the One who conquered death. In this Word are many promises: love, hope, forgiveness, and patience. He is rich in everything; all you need to do is ask for it.

You can believe what the Word says: *"And my God will meet all your needs according to the riches of his glory in Christ Jesus" (Philippians 4:19)* or *"All the prophets testify about him that everyone who believes in him receives forgiveness of sins through his name" (Acts 10:43).*

The more I read the Word of God and the more I meditated

on it, the more I felt my fear and depression melting away. So I started meditating on His Word on a daily basis, and it intensified my faith. This type of faith is a gift from God. Not everyone receives it, but because my heavenly Father loves me so much, He GAVE me this faith. This has got to be the most precious gift I have ever received in my life. Now, I could finally believe that I was forgiven—I could relate with the man who said, *"Blessed is the one whose transgressions are forgiven, whose sins are covered"* (Psalm 32:1).

I had the happiness of a lottery winner when I realized the freedom I was given and when I understood the gift that my Father was giving me. My burdens were becoming lighter and my fears were being removed. So rather than sitting around feeling sorry for myself and viewing myself as a disease-ridden person, I started taking on my regular chores with Holy Spirit gusto. I felt free to go to my heavenly Father with the things that weighed me down rather than expressing my concerns to all those around me. I also distanced myself from those who were faint hearted. I only liked to speak to those who were courageous and were unafraid to face difficult circumstances.

The Word of God, to me, seemed sweeter than honey. One day, my youngest daughter called from Chicago and spoke to my husband to see how I was doing. In a light-hearted response, my husband replied, "She's pregnant with the Word of God." His observation was correct; my mind was filled with words of hope. I felt like Jeremiah the prophet when he said, *"When your words came, I ate them; they were my joy and my heart's delight, for I bear your name, Lord God Almighty"* (Jeremiah 15:16). My Father in heaven wrote words of courage and hope in my heart. I felt as if He was speaking to me directly when I read from the book again: *"I have loved you with an everlasting love; I have drawn you with unfailing kindness"* (Jeremiah 31:3). My heart was brimming with love.

Then, I repented. I repented of four sins in particular:

1. For not believing the Word of God completely and wholeheartedly, even though I claimed to be a Christian
2. For desiring mercy from God but not always showing mercy toward others

3. For desiring forgiveness for my sins and transgression but not being able to forgive the sins and transgressions of others
4. For desiring love from God but not being willing to show that love to others

When I repented, God transformed me into a new person. I realized that I was not alone any longer, but that God who strengthened me would always be with me. I knew then that I did not need to be afraid of my cancer. Even Jesus felt the heaviness of carrying His cross and prayed to God that His cup could be removed. Carrying the cross is an impossible task, especially when you try to carry it yourself. God does not allow us to carry the cross ourselves; He did not allow Jesus to carry it by Himself as the book of Luke shows us: *An angel from heaven appeared to him and strengthened him (Luke 22:43).*

In the same way that God sustained Jesus Christ, I needed God to strengthen me because I realized the weakness of my flesh. I knew that I would not be able to face this journey alone. I knew that I needed God, and He was faithful to sustain me. Now, it became my responsibility to keep my heart pure and meditate daily on His Word because the proverb is true: *Above all else, guard your heart, for everything you do flows from it (Proverbs 4:23).*

Through repentance and meditation, the fear of death slowly faded away from my mind and the hope of salvation filled in its place. What a relief! I am no longer a slave to sin, but a child of the Most High—Jesus Christ.

> When we lose all that we hold dear (i.e. health, wealth), we become poor in spirit; it is this broken heart that builds a bridge to the heavens. God does not turn away any who approach Him with a despondent spirit. Instead, He fills us with the power and love of the Holy Spirit and we experience freedom from all that held us in chains. Later, I learned that I cannot control my thoughts in my own strength; for that, I would need grace from God, which is simply a gift to us from Him. Freedom from fear is the best gift that can be given to us.

A Child's Heart

When my youngest daughter was five years old, she believed very strongly in Santa Claus. One day in December, I wrapped up a gift to myself and put it under the Christmas tree with an inscription that said: "To Aley, From Santa." My daughter was filled with utter despair when she saw that the present was not for her, it was for me. Her innocent heart, so full of childlike faith, was filled with despair because she could not believe that Santa had left me a gift and none for her. Of course, today she practices as an attorney where facts are extremely important and where simple belief is completely out of the question. But at that time, when she was five years old, she believed.

That's what I asked for from God, to give me a childlike faith, one that believed wholeheartedly without any question. In the Word of God, there are many promises from my Father: healing, wisdom, love, and forgiveness. He made the lame walk and gave sight to the blind. He parted rivers and never condemned anyone. He gives courage in place of fear, replaces impossibility with possibility, turns our mourning into dancing, and shines light into the utter darkness of life. These are all promises that our heavenly Father gives:

- The blind will see
- The lame will walk
- Lepers will get healed
- The dead will rise
- The deaf will hear

These are not like human promises, which may or may not come to pass. God's promises stand true. They always come to pass regardless of race, denomination, or past sins. All that is required of us is a realization that we need His promises to come true in our life. We only need to be aware that we need the Holy Spirit to take away our fears, anxieties, and hopelessness. All I needed was to believe like a child and ask.

It was like the woman in the Bible who had been bleeding for twelve years. She had gone to every doctor in town and had tried every new tonic that was offered, but she still suffered from the same issue. She had tried everything, except Jesus. When He was on His way one day, she believed like a child.

She said to herself, "If I only touch his cloak, I will be healed" (Matthew 9:21).

She said to herself. She believed in her heart. She was convinced that Jesus could heal.

I imagined this scene in my head, and I put myself in the place of this woman. I saw myself reaching out to touch the hem of Jesus' cloak. I just knew that if I could touch His cloak, I would be healed. And I did it. With complete faith, I closed my eyes and reached out and received from Him.

John 5 tells the story of the man who had been disabled for thirty-eight years. He lay among other disabled people—the blind, the lame, and the paralyzed. They all lay there at Bethesda, a pool that was stirred by the Angel of God once a year. Whoever could reach the pool first would receive healing. This man had been there for thirty-eight years! When Jesus saw him lying there, He asked, "Do you want to get well?"

"Sir," the invalid replied, "I have no one to help me into the pool when the water is stirred. While I am trying to get in, someone else goes down ahead of me."

It was the same for me when I went to see the doctor. I went to UT Southwestern in Texas, a cancer center with a long-standing reputation for excellence. The waiting room was filled with cancer patients. Some were bold and others were shy. Some came with wigs and others came without. Some spoke freely about their disease and others kept quiet. Some saw it as a horrible disease and others saw it as a wave of the hand. I noticed all the differences, and I wished quietly that I could have the courage that the bold patients had. I wished that someone would be there to move me to a place of greater faith. I had the desire to be moved to a place of great faith and through that desire, the Lord provided. I began to believe that God would give it to me. I asked God in my helplessness to give me the Holy Spirit, and I believe that He gave me what I wanted; He gave me the Spirit of God. I had received the heart of a child. I was able to believe in His Word without any logical question. My faith was simple.

At that time Jesus said, "I praise you, Father, Lord of heaven and earth, because you have hidden these things from the wise and learned, and revealed them to little children" (Matthew 11:25).

God does not reside in an evil heart; rather, He resides in the heart of a child—in a pure heart. Guilt and thoughts of death will plague the mind, making the heart feel heavy and burdened. Search earnestly for courage, hope, and joy. Depraved thoughts come from an evil heart, so yearn for a pure heart, for it is the pure in heart who will see God.

Joshua told the people, "Consecrate yourselves, for tomorrow the Lord will do amazing things among you." (Joshua 3:5)

In the Bible during the time of Pharaoh's rule, the children of Israel groaned in their slavery and cried out to God to rescue them from the severe hands of Pharaoh. Hearing their painful pleas and because of their slavery, with mercy, the Lord was concerned. He sought out a man to deliver them—Moses, who was slow of speech and tongue—and pledged to bring them to the Promised Land, filled with milk and honey and freedom. However, to arrive at the Promised Land, they had to endure many challenges.

The Red Sea was probably the most difficult to overcome. A large, looming body of water lay out in front of them as they ran with all their might from the Egyptians who were chasing them. The answer for their dilemma was none other than the Holy Spirit. God told Moses to put his staff over the water and when he did, a mighty wind separated the waters into towering walls, which created a dry pathway for the Israelites to cross. The wind was the Holy Spirit. What was impossible in the eyes of man was possible by the might of the Holy Spirit.

Their next obstacle was the waters of Marah. They had been traveling for three days in the desert without water. The water in Marah was bitter, and they were thirsty and needed fresh water to drink. Although they had just experienced the miracle of the Red Sea three days prior, they grumbled and complained about the water. But

God heard their cries and offered yet another miracle. He told Moses to throw a piece of wood into the water, which caused the water to become fit to drink.

There were many challenges they had to face in the wilderness; there was no food, no water, there were discouraging thoughts, sickness, and strong desires to return back to Egypt. But God led them through each of their difficulties. He provided manna, brought forth water from a rock, and healed those who were sick. He delivered them even though they were rebellious. After forty years, when they were close to their destination, they faced yet another challenge; they had to cross the flooding waters of the Jordan.

Moses had already passed away and Joshua was leading the people. The Jordan looked like an impossible situation. But their fearless leader, Joshua, filled with faith, boldly told the people, *"Consecrate yourselves, for tomorrow the LORD will do amazing things among you."* Joshua instructed the priests, who carried the ark of the Lord, to enter the water first. When their feet touched the edge of the water, the rushing waters of the Jordan stopped flowing, and it piled up about a mile away upstream, allowing the entire nation of Israel to cross by on dry ground. What this teaches us is that there are a multitude of challenges as we travel to our promised land. But our Lord is able. He will not leave us in the middle of our struggles. We do not have to fear; He will lead us through. He will enable us to carry the burdens that need to be carried and will give us the Holy Spirit to strengthen us.

To determine whether my cancer was localized to the right breast only or whether it had spread to other parts of my body, I had to have a bone scan. When I arrived at the doctor's office for my bone scan, I recognized the secretary as a lady I knew. Seeing my diagnosis, she wrapped her arms around my neck and cried with hopeless tears. Seeing her state of mind, I became weak and restless. Soon, the technician came and injected a dye into my veins. A few hours later, my test would start, but because I was restless, my husband took me out in the hallway to take a walk to calm me down. It did not help because all I could think of was the secretary's cry of hopelessness, which removed any peace that was within me.

As I walked around, I asked God to strengthen me the way that He strengthened Jesus. When the time of the test was near, I went back to the testing office and lay on the table with anxiousness. I was worried if the cancer had spread. I still do not like to recall my feelings of fear and hopelessness. I meditated as I lay on the table. While waiting for the scan and thinking of the floodwaters of the Jordan, I suddenly felt that the cancer, which is a quick growing cell, was like a flood, and that it might have overflowed into the other parts of my body. The bone scan would show whether or not the cancer had spread. I was gripped with fear, but all of a sudden, to encourage me, my Father sent me His Word: *"Consecrate yourselves, for tomorrow the Lord will do amazing things among you" (Joshua 3:5).* The wonder was carried out by the priests who were given authority to stop the flooding waters of the Jordan. To STOP the flooding waters of the Jordan! The book of Joshua explains it this way:

> *Now the Jordan is at flood stage all during harvest. Yet as soon as the priests who carried the ark reached the Jordan and their feet touched the water's edge, the water from upstream stopped flowing. It piled up in a heap a great distance away, at a town called Adam in the vicinity of Zarethan, while the water flowing down to the Sea of the Arabah (that is, the Dead Sea) was completely cut off. So the people crossed over opposite Jericho (Joshua 3:15–16).*

When I heard the Word of the Lord, I believed that the power of the priest was in me. Immediately, I put my hand on my breast and commanded the cancer to stop. I had received courage. I had received faith. I commanded the cancer to stop.

Similarly, when I had to take an MRI, a great fear paralyzed me. Taking an MRI is a scary experience because you have to lie on a table in a tightly enclosed area for nearly forty-five minutes with a very loud buzzing sound ringing in your ears. During that time, I wondered whether or not the cancer had spread, and the thought of it spreading caused a distressing spirit to enter into my mind. But what was amazing was that during those forty-five minutes, God brought to my mind His Word from Psalm 91. The chapter was being recited in my mind over and over to the point where my fears were removed and calmness was given. In addition, I began to think and pray for a friend of mine who was also fighting cancer of a very grave degree.

When I entered the MRI unit, I was fearful and anxious, but when I came out of it, God gave me courage and hope. The difference was so obvious that the MRI technician commented that my face was glowing after the MRI, which is certainly not common.

After Job had prayed for his friends, the LORD restored his fortunes and gave him twice as much as he had before (Job: 42:10).

When I stopped focusing on my needs and started praying for my friend instead, I received twice as much of a blessing.

To find out the result of the bone scan, I had to wait for two days. During my period of waiting, my surgeon, Dr. Roshni Rao, called me, and I picked up the phone with much anxiousness. What would the doctor say? Was the cancer localized or had it spread to other parts? I was anxious. Then Dr. Rao simply stated that the cancer had not spread and that it was local to my breast. When I heard the good news, I jumped up and down with joy. In my home, I gave thanks to my surgeon and to God and prayed yet again to God.

However, after the phone conversation and after my prayer, the devil of doubt quickly entered my mind, and I began to wonder whether or not I had heard the doctor correctly. Was the cancer in fact localized or had it spread? So I picked up the phone and called the surgeon back to ask her for confirmation of the results. Was she sure that the cancer had not spread? Did I hear correctly? She repeated to me that the cancer was localized and that I *did* hear correctly.

In 2 Kings chapter 5, it tells of the story of Naaman, the commander of the army of the king of Aram. Though he was a valiant soldier, Naaman suffered from leprosy. He desperately wanted to be healed. A young girl was taken captive during one of his raids and served as a maid to his wife. She told her mistress about Elisha, the prophet from Samaria who could certainly heal Naaman. When he heard of the possibility and went to Samaria to meet Elisha, divinely knowing about Naaman's visit, Elisha sent one of his servants to greet him. The servant asked him to go and dip himself in the rivers of the Jordan seven times for his flesh to be restored and for him to be cleansed. Naaman was not happy about the instructions that Elisha gave, but still he went and washed himself and he was healed. This miracle brought Naaman to faith. He believed after his healing that there was no God in the entire world except the God of Israel—so faith and obedience must come before healing.

Sanctification is the process of cleansing yourself. Before the Israelites crossed the rushing waters of the Jordan, they were told to sanctify themselves. Before Naaman could be healed, he was told to wash himself in the waters of the Jordan. Sanctification always comes before healing. Sanctification always comes before fear can be washed away; it is the key to receiving strength. Hearing the Word of God leads us to faith, faith leads to sanctification, and sanctification delivers us from our weaknesses. It replaces misery with hope and restores joy. It relieves dependency on people and shifts that dependency to God. When we are sanctified, God resides in our hearts. No longer are we on our own. The One who bore the great cross inhabits our hearts and makes it possible for us to endure our own crosses, and He relieves our fear of death. Instead, we are able to receive the promise of eternity in heaven.

When I first received the news of my cancer, I was paralyzed with fear. I was not ready to meet my Creator. I was not ready to face judgment. The thought of death crippled me. My cries to God were from utter desperation. From the agony in my belly, I wailed unto God. It was a plea and not a request. It came from the anguish in my soul. It was this soul-bearing humility that created an atmosphere for desire. From desire was created an ear to hear the Word of God and a heart to receive the Word of God. So as God whispered His promises to me, He began to sanctify me. I heard the Word of God, I received the Word of God, and He started to cleanse me. I did nothing to deserve it. I felt that I was being washed and made pure. This was my sanctification. It relieved me from my fears. It enabled me to endure my cross. It caused me to accept the promise of eternity in heaven. I was overjoyed!

When raw, tough meat is put into a pressure cooker, it

becomes soft and tender. In the same way, I believe that God put pressure on me to soften my heart. I believe today that God resides in my heart.

But he knows the way that I take; when he has tested me, I will come forth as gold (Job 23:10).

God, filled with mercy, calls everyone to this salvation, not just me.

May God himself, the God of peace, sanctify you through and through. May your whole spirit, soul and body be kept blameless at the coming of our Lord Jesus Christ (1 Thessalonians 5:23).

Therefore, since we have these promises, dear friends, let us purify ourselves from everything that contaminates body and spirit, perfecting holiness out of reverence for God (2 Corinthians 7:1).

When I had unbelief in my heart, I lived with fear, hopelessness, and anxiety. What a great sin is unbelief! Faith is tested when the great challenges of life are presented before us. Through this sickness of cancer, Jesus Christ called me into His holiness. From this trial, I was born again. Like a newborn child who is delivered through pain is this newfound faith of mine. Though it was painful to endure, it was soon forgotten because what was newly born brought so much joy, and no one can steal this joy from me. The book of John explains it well:

A woman giving birth to a child has pain because her time has come; but when her baby is born she forgets the anguish because of her joy that a child is born into the world. So with you: Now is your time of grief, but I will see you again and you will rejoice, and no one will take away your joy. In that day you will no longer ask me anything. Very truly I tell you, my Father will give you whatever you ask in my name (John 16:21–23).

Rather than focusing on the existing sickness or failure and allowing it to birth fear and disappointment, look *hopefully* toward the good things that God has in store for your future. The Lord has promised that His blessings will come, even if there is a delay. Intensify your thoughts toward the promises—this is how to free yourself from perilous feelings.

Strength to Triumph over the Fiery Trial

$\mathcal{I}$ called my family in India to inform them of my sickness; I have five brothers, one sister, and a mother. Upon hearing the terrible news, all of them cried helplessly. They could not accept the fact and had no words of hope to offer. But the brother to whom I was closest and who also had gone through heavy trials himself found words of hope to encourage me and to give me a new perspective to my situation. Using my pet name he said, "Ponnamma, this is nothing but a tiny scab." About ten years ago, he had endured hemorrhaging and went into a coma for some time. His healing was miraculous because one day, even though no anecdote had been prescribed, the doctors could see no more bleeding. He reminded me of his victory over his own horrific experiences. Even though he walked through the valley of the shadow of death, he experienced God's protection and favor. My brother knew that God was the only one who could strengthen me.

The Bible tells the story of three young men who were thrown in a fiery pit by the king because they would not worship the gods or the images of gold that the king had set up. Shadrach, Meshach, and Abednego were men of faith who believed and trusted in their Lord their God and were not easily frightened by the king's punishment. They told the king, "King Nebuchadnezzar, we do not need to defend ourselves before you in this matter. If we are thrown into the blazing furnace, the God we serve is able to deliver us from it, and he will deliver us from Your Majesty's hand. But even if he does not, we want you to know, Your Majesty, that we will not serve your gods or worship the image of gold you have set up" (Daniel 3:16–18).

So, King Nebuchadnezzar, raging with anger that his authority was not revered, threw them into the furnace and ordered it to be heated seven times hotter than normal. So these men, wearing their robes, trousers, turbans, and other clothes, were bound and thrown into the blazing furnace. The king's command was so urgent and the furnace so hot that the flames of the fire killed the soldiers who took up Shadrach, Meshach, and Abednego, and these three men, firmly tied, fell into the blazing furnace (Daniel 3:21–23).

Though he watched with anticipation and expected the men to burn to ashes, to the king's amazement, he suddenly saw four men walking unbound and unharmed around the fire! He said, "Look! I see four men walking around in the fire, unbound and unharmed, and the fourth looks like a son of the gods" (Daniel 3:25). He went to the opening of the furnace and ordered the men to come out.

So Shadrach, Meshach, and Abednego came out of the fire, and the satraps, prefects, governors, and royal advisers crowded around them. They saw that the fire had not harmed their bodies, nor was a hair of their heads singed; their robes were not scorched, and there was no smell of fire on them (Daniel 3:26–27).

When we are put through fiery trials, all we need to do is put our faith in God. He will unchain us, walk beside us, and pour out His power on us. Only when we are in the middle of a fire do we realize our need and become desperate for God. In that desperation, we are able to see things more clearly and we are able to receive revelation. Only then can we open up the Bible and see the words of God come to life. Only then do we have a yearning for God's deliverance and nothing else. So, just like a seed that is planted and develops deep roots, these fiery trials help our faith to take root. It is the trial that pushes us (forces us) to rely on God with excessive desperation and brings us to a place of incredible growth.

Another story in the Bible speaks of a woman whose eyes were opened to a miracle but only when she was at a place of desperation. Her name was Hagar, and she was the slave of Abraham and Sarah. She was given to Abraham by Sarah to conceive a child. After that child was born, Sarah also conceived a boy—Isaac. When Isaac was of a certain age, Sarah did not like the fact that her son had to abide with her slave's son, so she asked Abraham to send Hagar and her son away. With approval from God, Abraham put Hagar out. As she walked through the heat of the desert with her child, she ran out of water. With fear and anguish in her heart, she put her child under a bush, walked a few feet away, and began to sob heavily. In the midst of her extreme anxiety, an angel approached her with words of hope saying that God would make her child into a great nation. Then, he opened her eyes and she saw a well of water.

Only in a place of desperation can our eyes be opened to see what God has placed before us. These kinds of trials will open our eyes. These trials are our training ground to prepare us for doing God's work. To work for the Lord requires patience, love, compassion, and courage. When we endure the trial, we develop these skills.

Blessed is the one who perseveres under trial because, having stood the test, that person will receive the crown of life that the Lord has promised to those who love him (James 1:12).

Because of my trials, my thinking started to gradually change. I started to believe that my cancer could be completely removed through surgery and treatment. The cancer was only temporary and not life threatening. My doctor advised me to have a mastectomy done (complete removal of the right breast). Before I went into surgery—and to get more medical advice—I took my medical report to the pathologist who worked with me, Dr. Beverly Rogers. After reading my report, she helped me to better understand the situation. She explained that the cancer had escaped through the ducts in my breast and was not contained within. In other words, it was not ductal carcinoma in situ (DCIS); rather, it was Invasive Ductal Carcinoma (IDC).

IDC is a very common type of breast cancer. It starts developing in the milk ducts of the breast, but breaks out of the duct tubes and invades, or infiltrates, surrounding tissues. Unlike DCIS, which is a noninvasive cancer, IDC is not a well-contained cancer. IDC has the potential to invade your lymph and blood systems, spreading cancer cells to other parts of your body. If IDC spreads beyond its original site, it has metastasized.[1]

[1] Pam Stephan, "Invasive Ductal Carcinoma—IDC Breast

The Audacious Dr. Rogers

After Dr. Rogers explained the invasiveness of my cancer, she hugged me and to my utter shock, she asked me, "Why don't you take leadership of the microbiology lab?" I had been working at Children's Medical Center as a medical technologist for the past twenty years; I had never taken on any leadership roles. I was a worker bee, not a queen.

When I first went to Dr. Rogers, I thought she would sympathize with my situation, but instead she saw an opportunity in the midst of my struggle. At first, I could not understand where her mindset was, and I did not like that she tried to challenge me rather than offering me her pity. When I came home, I pondered over the conversation and wondered why she said something like that to me; wasn't it rude for her to say that to me?

Then my thinking suddenly changed. Since she was a pathologist and director of the labs at Children's Medical Center, I realized that despite the demands of her position, she pushed herself to take further responsibilities in other hospitals as well. She found opportunity in the midst of difficulty. I remembered the verse that says: Then the LORD God formed a man from the dust of the ground and breathed into his nostrils the breath of life, and the man became a living being (Genesis 2:7). I concluded that I, too, had the breath of God inside of me, which was powerful enough to prevail over this fiery trial. This Spirit that is spoken of here is omnipresent; it is able to strengthen us at any time. The Spirit has no kind of sickness, the Spirit has no death, and the Spirit connects us to eternity in heaven. When we come to an awareness of this Spirit living inside of us, we can transform our tests and trials into opportunities. When we are cognizant that the Holy Spirit of God lives inside of us, we start to alleviate our fears. I thank God that He has given me this gift—to have this kind of awareness and to receive this kind of faith.

Cancer," American Cancer Society, April 1, 2011; (accessed via Web site About.com, 27 January 2011.)

When my director encouraged me to take on more responsibilities, she pushed me to take risks and that brought fear. I realized it was the fear that made me dislike her coercion, and I knew that I would have to break that fear if I was to do anything productive in my life. I realized I would have to move from my comfort zone and into a faith zone. I knew that move would be difficult. But I knew that if I moved, it would only bring about a healthy conversion, which would ultimately bring joy and livelihood.

The man who invented the light bulb, Thomas Edison, did not live a life devoid of calamity. In fact, he lost his hearing at a young age and was deaf for the larger part of his living years. But he never allowed the hearing loss to handicap him, and he did not end up on welfare; in fact, he went on to create over a thousand patents in his name and is known as the fourth most productive inventor in history.

My own mother also, due to typhoid fever, lost her hearing during her middle age. But she never complained about it; in fact, she has said that she was glad to have lost her hearing so that she did not have to listen to undesirable things around her. My mother is a very spiritual lady, and I know that it was the Holy Spirit that enabled her to consider her hearing loss as an advantage in life rather than a handicap. She always found ways to help those less fortunate and gave an abundance of love to all those around her. She was known in her community as a generous lady—in spirit and in goods.

There are some who, like Edison and my mother, do not allow their weaknesses to make them a burden to others; instead, they find ways to bring about good and benefit society. Meanwhile, there are those who fall prey to victim thinking and become an inconvenience to society. I knew that Dr. Rogers was trying to pull me out of my own state of helplessness and to push past my feelings of self-pity. It was a choice I had to make—remain pathetic or become worthwhile.

One day as I was waiting for my surgery, I remembered a story I had read a long time ago.

The mother somehow passed away. No one knew where the father was. The baby lion was alone. Along his way came a herd of sheep. With joy, the baby lion joined the herd. Poor baby lion, he had no one. The herd of sheep took pity upon the baby lion. The sheep told the lion to join them. In that way, the baby lion became a part of the sheep herd and grew with them. He had no idea who he was. He did not know the strength that a lion should have, and no one told him that he was a child of the king of the jungle. Walking with the sheep and eating their grub of leaves, the baby lion lived. He baaed like a sheep and kept a quiet personality, much like the sheep. The baby lion thought he was a sheep.

One day, another lion stalked the sheep from a mountaintop far away, and he noticed that among the sheep herd was a baby lion. So he looked a second time carefully and verified that it was in fact a baby lion, and he roared. The baby lion looked back and saw a creature that looked exactly like himself, and observed his impressive, majestic presence. So the baby lion cried back in a tiny voice, and he comprehended that he also was an impressive, majestic creature. He quickly ran away from the sheep herd and joined the herd of lions.

This baby lion represents many of us. Not knowing our identity or the strengths and capabilities that lie with us, we exist as that baby lion that lived among a herd of sheep. When we understand that we are a child of the Almighty God, only then can we embrace who we truly are. Only then can we receive ten-fold more strength than what we believe we have. Only when we look up to our Maker do we recognize whose image we are made in.

Around this time, I remembered an Indian Christian song that spoke to the human consciousness by saying something like: "Hold still. Do not forget about the God who makes all things possible. God will honor you and give you a spirit of boldness and replace your hesitations with fearlessness" (paraphrased). As I listened and focused on the words of this song, I stopped being uncertain and reluctant and started getting excited about how God would honor me. I understood that everything I would have to go through with surgery and chemo was only temporary, but my future held an exciting possibility.

It is not the enemy outside of us that we need to be afraid of, rather it is the enemy within. Our own enemies take on various forms: lack of confidence, sadness, dissatisfaction, complaints, doubt, inadequate feelings, insecurity, and anger linger within. We must acquire a desire to get victory over these enemies. We must conquer our negative emotions with God's strength.

We demolish arguments and every pretension that sets itself up against the knowledge of God, and we take captive every thought to make it obedient to Christ (2 Corinthians 10:5).

The Beginning of Transformation

I decided that I wanted to get control over my negative thoughts. The Word of God gives thoughts of hope and courage; they are positive, not negative. The apostle Paul said when we are weak, He is strong. God expects me to live victoriously. I want to be a victor, not a victim. I made up my mind that I would fight against the sickness and against my negative thoughts. This trial is a test of my faith. I told myself, "Don't give up! Don't quit. Don't complain. Don't ask God why is this happening to me? Instead, stand strong and fight the good fight of faith." Like my pathologist told me, I would take this as an opportunity for promotion, and an opportunity to take on more responsibility. Then God blessed me with the passage of 1 Samuel 17, the story of David and Goliath.

Goliath was a giant, larger than everyone around him. He was so physically strong that the very armor he wore seemed to be heavier than what most men could barely carry, and this giant challenged the Israelites to send a man to fight him. Now, David was just a small shepherd boy who tended sheep, and his father sent him out to see how his brothers were doing. As he was speaking to his brothers, he heard the challenge that Goliath roared out. So David stepped forward. Even his brothers did not like it. King Saul discouraged him saying that he was just a little boy and that he would not be able to defeat Goliath. But David never gave up. He had experience, a desert experience where with the help of God, he was able to kill a lion and a bear with his bare hands. So he believed that he could defeat Goliath. David said, "The Lord who rescued me from the paw of the lion and the paw of the bear will rescue me from the hand of this Philistine" (1 Samuel 17:37). David believed that his defeat was not because of his physical strength or because of his smart wit; rather it was because of God's power.

Through this story, God reaffirmed the things that I was learning. He showed me how there would always be giants in my life—great obstacles to overcome—and He reminded me that He would deliver me through every one of those difficulties. During my days of childhood and youth, I never experienced hardship, and I desired only comfort; however, I had no idea that my adult life would be filled with difficulties, but nothing so hard that I should fear. Rather, the giants in my life could be overcome. I would have to fight, but I knew that with God, I would win. There was no fear of failure. I desired only to win. My mind was being transformed. I understood now what Paul meant when he said, "I can do all things through him who gives me strength" (Philippians 4:13).

In a similar manner, the book of Jeremiah tells the story of Jeremiah who was sent by God to the potter's house so that he could illustrate God's ultimate rein.

This is the word that came to Jeremiah from the LORD: "Go down to the potter's house, and there I will give you my message." So I went down to the potter's house, and I saw him working at the wheel. But the pot he was shaping from the clay was marred in his hands; so the potter formed it into another pot, shaping it as seemed best to him (Jeremiah 18:1–4).

Pots are fashioned by using only pliable material, clay, and by heating them to extremely high temperatures. The supple nature of clay allows it to be kneaded and shaped. A process called firing applies temperatures between the ranges of 1000 to 1400°C and produces irreversible changes in the body. It is only after firing that the clay can be considered pottery. If the clay is not put through the fire, it will not harden; it will break.

In the same way, when people are put through fiery trials, many want to give up and turn away. Some become depressed, others become angry, others isolate themselves, and some commit suicide. But those who maintain hope, desire to be a new vessel, and surrender to God will be given strength. They will be fashioned into a beautiful pot, and they will not break. But the choice is ours. We have to surrender. Pride must be thrown out the door and we must realize that only Christ has the authority. When the fires are thrown our way, we must learn how to dream within its crux. We must be able to envision ourselves as new vessels in the midst of our fiery trial because the fires are God's way of testing us and changing us.

What a privilege to be chosen by God in this manner to be formed by Him!

You did not choose me, but I chose you and appointed you so that you might go and bear fruit—fruit that will last—and so that whatever you ask in my name the Father will give you (John 15:16).

When you come to a strong faith in God, you will no longer fear the difficult challenges that life throws your way. Instead, you will always see an opportunity; this perspective removes hopelessness. When dark forces attack us, rather than falling prey, we must look them boldly in the face and fight because the One who is higher than them is with us. Perseverance, which is a gift from God, must accompany the trials in life, for it is through the trial that God chooses us for greater dominion.

Mastectomy, My Pruning

My surgeon, Dr. Rao, recommended a mastectomy, removal of the breast, as the best treatment for my condition. I believed it to be one of the most important organs on a woman's body, and it would have to be removed from mine. I considered having a lumpectomy. With a lumpectomy, only the cancerous lump would have to be removed and not the entire breast. I was mentally anguished because I did not want any part of the cancer left in my body, but I also did not want to lose the most feminine organ on me. How embarrassed would I feel in front of my husband? I would have to face pain on two different levels—the physical pain of surgery and the mental agony of living the rest of my life with a flattened chest. I thought about how carefully I had designed sari blouses in the past to flatter my figure, but with the mastectomy, I would have to let go of the pride I took in my body's appearance. Never in my life did I ever think that I would end up without a breast.

Because so much development and research has been put into breast cancer here in America, many organizations have participated to help cancer patients. One such organization was purporting a "look good, feel good" campaign aimed at providing patients with cancer-safe cosmetics, wigs, and application training. I had no desire to go, but my daughter pushed me to attend. They taught me how to apply my makeup and my wig, among other things. While I was there, I realized that even though I would lose a breast, I could get an artificial one that looked very similar to the real thing. Rather than giving too much importance to this physical aspect, I spent more of my focus making sure my mind would be stable.

I was scared to have the surgery. I remembered when I had my uterus removed. The surgery came in the same year that I had a seizure, but it came after the seizure. The hysterectomy led to an infection and pain. It was a very uncomfortable experience.

During a mastectomy when biopsying the sentinel node, a pathologist can determine whether or not the cancer has spread. This will also allow the doctor to determine the grade of the cancer—G1 being the lowest and G4 being the highest. My tumor was graded at G2, intermediate grade.

Before the surgery, my feelings were like a roller coaster; they would go up and down. I felt anxiety and all sorts of negative emotions. The night before the surgery, my priest and some family and friends gathered at my home to pray for me and to strengthen my spirits. But nothing they said or did gave me comfort or strength. I had to go into my prayer closet and meditate on my own because that was how I gained strength in the past. The night before the surgery, I meditated on my own. During that time of prayer, God gave me a Word from John 15:2: *"He cuts off every branch in me that bears no fruit, while every branch that does bear fruit he prunes so that it will be even more fruitful."*

Pruning is painful, but the good news is that after the pruning, there are beautiful blossoms and ripe, delicious fruit. God chose me, and I had to accept that pain in order to gain something great. I had to go through this mastectomy as a part of my pruning. God had to prune the cancer from my body and from my mind, and when He did so, I would be ready to bring forth new blossoms, cancer free.

"I am the true vine, and my Father is the gardener. He cuts off every branch in me that bears no fruit, while every branch that does bear fruit he prunes so that it will be even more fruitful" (John 15:1–2).

My heavenly Father put me into a family that was blessed. They were disciplined people; they knew God, and they were wise in their ways. I never faced any hardships growing up. I was given a good education and was provided with all sorts of opportunities, but I did not take anything seriously. My mother was, and remains, a religious lady. I have heard it said that she fasted and prayed for my conception. She was joyful in helping the poor. I knew that I had my mother's heart, but I was a bit lazy. I preferred to live in comfort and not worry too much about my neighbor. I had a desire to help cancer patients, but it remained only a desire; I never did anything about it. God knew my heart because He's the One who gave me this passion. I believe that He put me through these difficult situations to gain a heart of understanding. Because I was lazy and selfish, not only was I not very fruitful, the meager fruits that I did produce were sour and not sweet. I did not meet my Father's expectations, and so He decided to prune me to get more and better fruit out of me. These were the thoughts that ran through my head the night before.

The next morning, my family brought me to the hospital where I would receive my surgery. At the hospital, they injected a radioactive substance around the tumor followed by a blue dye. They then tracked the dye and identified the sentinel lymph node. My family and friends were with me while I received this injection and they were all crying. When I saw them crying, I felt my courage draining away. Prior to this moment, my mind was filled with all that God had planned for my future, and I was excited that I would receive a cancer-free body and cancer-free thoughts. My conscience had forgotten about the surgery. But when I saw my friends and family crying, my anxieties came back, and I thought about the women who mourned and wailed over Jesus being seized by the soldiers. Jesus' response to them was *"Daughters of Jerusalem, do not weep for me; weep for yourselves and for your children" (Luke 23:28)*. Jesus knew that after the cross, there would be resurrection. The cross was temporary, but it was difficult. But He had no choice; He had to take the cross to experience the resurrection. An angel from heaven strengthened Christ, but He had to endure the cross. In the same way, I knew I would have to carry my cross, but I wouldn't be able to carry it on my own. I knew I would receive strength from above to carry my cross. When I received this thought, I was able to take the injection with courage.

They then took me to the operation theater, a place where none of my family or friends was allowed. In that room, I had no one to turn to; only one person was allowed to come into that area with me—Jesus Christ, my Father in heaven. His presence can go with us everywhere; He is not limited by "Do Not Enter" signs. There is a limit to man's bounty because he is finite, so it is best not to put your hope on him. So I lay there with Christ alone.

Before the surgery, the anesthesiologist and the surgeon came to me, and anxiety settled in. Prior to the surgery, my children had extensively researched the surgeon, her credentials, and her credibility. It was important to my family to have confidence in the surgeon, but life experience reminded me that even she, with all her experience and education, could make mistakes. Man is imperfect; he can err. An organ would be removed from my body, and if my surgeon made one slight mistake, it would affect my body for the rest of my life. Even though my surgeon was not Christian and practiced Hinduism, I asked her if it would be okay to pray with her. She respected my beliefs and faith and agreed. I held her hands and prayed that the One who is capable would make her capable as well; that her hands would be guided by Him alone. In the same way, I held hands with the anesthesiologist and prayed. My anxieties and nervousness left, and I was wheeled to the operation room with courage. When my surgery was complete, my anesthesiologist told me something interesting. He gave me the anesthesia and as I entered into unconsciousness, I said to him, "God sent an angel to me."

After the surgery, everyone commented on how my face was glowing. Rather than looking weak and tired, it looked fresh and alive. God gave me the strength to handle the pain and discomfort. The area of my body that had the cancer was removed. I was no longer a cancer patient; I was cancer free. My Strengthener, through my surgeon's hands, pruned me and cut off that defective area. My right breast had been removed.

In the same way that an employer has expectations of his employees and parents have expectations of their children, God has expectations of His creation. God expects good fruit and will prune those who are not producing. Though it is painful, it is necessary. But through the pruning, your life will be transformed into one of significance and you will come to appreciate the pruning.

Chemotherapy, the Frightening Monster

I witnessed firsthand the suffering my father endured during his treatment of cancer. Regarding chemotherapy, I had an utter dread. The foreboding over the chemo was even stronger than I had for the actual cancer itself. The doctor educated me on the side effects of chemo:

> Within a few days: Nausea, vomiting, fatigue, allergic reaction
>
> Delayed side effects within a few weeks/month: Hair loss, low blood count, which may cause infection and even death, numbness and tingling in the fingers and toes
>
> Long term, after several years: Leukemia, memory loss, cloudy thinking, and infertility

I had a lot of anxiety. I saw chemo as an anaconda opening wide its mouth to swallow me whole.

When I was about thirteen years old and living in India something horrible happened. Before I explain what happened, I have to explain how houses were built in that time. All of our homes—mine and all of my relatives—were built with barred windows that had no netting and no glass. India is a very hot place, and air conditioners were not a common commodity in the homes in the 1960s, so windows were built as open spaces to allow airflow.

My uncle's house was in the process of being built. A portion of it was completed, but another part of it was left to be built. My cousins, who were twelve and eight, shared one bed in this open home. One particular night when the rains were heavy, a poisonous snake crawled in through the open window into their bed and bit both of them, killing two innocent lives on one dreary night. No one knew the children had been bitten when they woke up in the middle of the night asking to go to the restroom. After seeing the children become nauseated, vomit, and go through many horrible symptoms, they assumed the children had been poisoned. With no infrastructure in place for ambulances and emergency care, they called on a man who knew how to treat poison. But by the time the man arrived at their home on that rainy night, my eight-year-old cousin had already died. When he examined them, he saw that their ears and jawbone had turned black from poison and was able to deduce that the children had been bitten by a venomous snake. Sadly, before the family could even start a journey to the hospital, the older daughter also died. From that moment on, I was terrified of snakes. A seed of fear had been planted.

In 1980, after getting a C-section for my second daughter, Benji, while lying on the hospital bed in Thiruvilla Medical Mission Hospital in Kerala, India, I could hear the loud painful cries of a young girl in ICU. When the nurse came to my bedside, I asked what was wrong with the young girl. The nurse told me that a snake had bitten her. How painful is the venom of a snake! The seed of fear was being watered.

It was only about thirty-two years later when I was diagnosed with cancer that I realized that the small seed of fear had grown into an uncontrollable pasture of overgrown weeds that were now ready to choke me to death.

I began to think that chemotherapy was a poison; similar to a snake's venom, it is a chemical poison. It kills healthy cells along with cancer cells. Cancer cells divide more quickly than normal cells. Cells that divide quickly are easily damaged or destroyed. Chemo works because even though it does affect some normal cells, it kills the quickly dividing cancer cells as well.[2]

[2] Sharon Sorensen and Suzanne Metzger, *The Complete Idiot's Guide to Living with Breast Cancer,* (Indianapolis: Alpha Books), 2000.

Chemotherapy is a chemical poison. It would destroy the good cells in my body, and it would cause my hair to fall out. This was the poison that would be injected into my veins through the IV. Anxiety and sorrow settled in my soul. With my right breast already removed, the thought of losing all my hair brought additional despair. The more distressed I felt on the inside, the weaker I felt physically. So I prayed yet again to God, "Lord, You had blessed me with Your Word in every instance up to this point." Because all the side effects were so clearly communicated to us, our entire family felt we needed to prepare for a disaster. The house was cleaned, buckets were bought to contain the upcoming vomit, and cancer-safe lotions were purchased. My family took every care to prepare for my comfort, but they could not carry my sorrow and apprehension so I had to rely yet again on meditation. Praise God because He sent a great Word to strengthen me, but it did more; it spoke so acutely to the exact fear I held. This was the Word:

"I have given you authority to trample on snakes and scorpions and to overcome all the power of the enemy; nothing will harm you" (Luke 10:19).

Even though the doctor told me that there would be immediate, delayed, and long-term side effects, my heavenly Father said that I would not endure anything that I could not handle. Jesus did not just claim this for the seventy disciples; He gave this power to me as well because when He created me, He breathed His Holy Spirit into me. I am from a royal family! The royal blood of Jesus is the blood that runs through my veins. In that way, I convinced myself that not only would I not be harmed by the side effects, but I would be given dominion over these effects. So with courage, my family and I went off to get my first round of chemo at the oncology clinic.

The oncologist, Dr. Jenny Li, after reading the side effects that included possible death, made me sign the forms. The American system, unlike that in India, requires the doctor to inform the patient of everything that will happen to him/her. Only after acknowledging a comprehension of the procedure and signing the form are you allowed to proceed with the therapy. I felt like a sheep that was being taken to the slaughter. I was brought to the treatment room. I was given a hug. I was told not to be afraid. I let them know that all my fears were gone. God had given me a Word and strengthened me. I told the doctor that I was given authority to trample on snakes and scorpions and to overcome all the power of the enemy; nothing would harm me. I told the doctor that her patients who come here for treatment come with a lot of fear and that she needed to share that Word with those people.

Before the chemotherapy was applied, the nausea medicine was first injected through the IV into my veins. While the injections were given, I listened to very hopeful music through my headphones. The chemo drugs, Taxotere and Cytoxin, were then injected into my veins. As I sat there listening to the music, my mind began to imagine that power was running through my veins. I believed that I had royal blood, the blood of Jesus that was more powerful than the drugs, flowing through my veins. In my head, with much valor, I commanded the drugs to not touch my good cells and to only kill the cancerous cells. I believed that is exactly what would happen. Once the IV was completed, I went home with tenacity in my step.

The next morning, Dr. Li called me to find out if I had suffered any immediate side effects. I was able to respond that I did not suffer any nausea, vomiting, or fatigue because of the grace of God. But I knew I would lose my hair, and I prepared mentally for that time. That's when I came across the most interesting story of the eagle's rebirth.

Although the validity of this story is questionable, it points out an important lesson.

This is a story of the eagle's life.

The eagle is the most majestic bird in the sky, but something happens to all eagles at least once in their lifetime—they molt. In the life of every eagle, they will go through a molting process that can bring with it a great depression. Certain eagles live for about thirty years or more, but then they begin to lose their feathers. Their beaks and claws begin to alter as well. The eagle will walk and they have no strength at all to fly. The molting eagle finds himself in the valley, unable to fly, with its feathers falling out. They lose their ability to see, as well; their vision weakens during this time. They lose their desire to eat. They only eat fresh meat, but they have no strength to hunt. Now at this time, they will choose some area of a mountain range where the sun can shine directly on them, and they will lie on a rock and bathe in the sun. Some have observed other eagles coming and dropping food to the ones going through this "molting" stage. Yet it is never the younger eagles that drop the food; it is always the older eagles that have survived this experience and know what the molting eagle is going through. If they don't renew, they will die. They grow weaker and weaker. Suddenly, there comes a sound from the sky over the valley. Screaming loudly, a group of eagles fly overhead and drop fresh meat over the dying birds. The screaming is encouragement. That's what they reckon; the screaming is encouragement from other eagles who have already gone through this. Some eat and recover, but others roll over and die. Don't you think all of this speaks of something in our Christian lives as well?

Just like the eagle lost everything—its feathers, its claws, its beak, and its pride—the chemo patient also loses everything and is brought down low. Some eagles stay in the valley while others fly toward the sun. Some patients, in a similar manner, will not stay in their valley; they will rise up and take flight. It is the older eagles who have survived their state of molting who bring food for the eagles who are going through their own experience. In the same way, cancer survivors brought me "food for thought." The survivors knew the valley experience, and they could provide a glimmer of hope.

Chemotherapy brings with it a time of mourning; it is a time of loneliness, withdrawal, and devastation. The physical wreckage (like the loss of hair, loss of appetite, loss of weight) of the therapy brought a feeling of intense helplessness. It stripped me of any pride that I held and replaced it with a humiliating awareness of my own weakness. It was during the time of chemotherapy that I learned to depend solely on the Word of God. I read with hunger and it satiated my soul. One story that spoke to me was the story of Elijah's fear. Elijah was a great prophet of God who was given many revelations and performed great miracles. He walked with the strength of God, yet when his enemy pursued him, he fled with fear and with anguish cried unto God to take his life. However, God touched him, gave him nourishment, and encouraged him to continue his journey. In the same way, when I became weak, God touched me, gave me nourishment, and encouraged me to continue my journey because I had many things left to accomplish.

But blessed is the one who trusts in the Lord, whose confidence is in him. They will be like a tree planted by the water that sends out its roots by the stream. It does not fear when heat comes; its leaves are always green. It has no worries in a year of drought and never fails to bear fruit (Jeremiah 17:7–8).

In the same way that the eagle renews itself, I became renewed. But it wasn't just new hair that I received; rather, it was a new mindset, the ability to look fear in its face and claim victory, and the command to handle great responsibility. Even though I began this journey seeing chemotherapy as a monster, I am now able to see that the supreme God is much bigger.

He gives strength to the weary and increases the power of the weak. Even youths grow tired and weary, and young men stumble and fall; but those who hope in the Lord will renew their strength. They will soar on wings like eagles; they will run and not grow weary, they will walk and not be faint (Isaiah 40:29–31).

To battle the crisis that surely comes in everyone's life, we must cry out to God morning and night and let Him know that we are weak not just in body but also in mind. We should not presume that man can encourage us, for man is not equipped to help us in our time of distress and weakness. Even the most capable will get worn out after some time. However, our limitless God knows no bounds in providing strength for the weak hearted or peace for the desolate. The weak and strong alike have God.

My first day back at work while being treated with chemo

In between my chemotherapy sessions, I went back to work. I work as a microbiologist in a medical lab dealing with bacteria, where my body could easily catch infection. I decided to work on the weekends when there were fewer people and I could take my time to do my work. When my director heard that I was coming to work, she met me there on a weekend with a card and flowers. My co-workers welcomed me with love and joy. I sat at my desk and began my work. My work requires a lot of focused attention, but my eyes started wandering. I began to notice that everyone else around me was well, but I was the only sick person. I was also working with a wig on my head and a mask on my face. I began to feel sorry for myself and suddenly felt intolerable pain and the tears began to overflow.

I quickly left the lab to go into an empty room so that no one would see my tears, and I wiped my eyes. I felt my strength draining, and I realized that I may not be able to do my work. I picked up the phone and called a friend of mine, Lizy, and told her, "Lizy, I cannot handle the pain in my heart; I have no strength in me to contain my emotion much less do my work." I asked her to sing a song with me. The words of the song said, "O Holy Spirit, bestow your strength upon me, I need the power of your spirit that flows from you, I need it. Oh! God, you know I need your help, please do not take your Holy Spirit from me." Just then, God strengthened me again. It did not matter that I had only one breast; America has plenty of plastic surgeons who could reconstruct it. To cover up my hair loss, I could get a really nice wig with great style. I could use makeup to cover my skin that was being affected. Everything external could be replaced. But if I lost my mind, I would not be able to do anything

It was my responsibility to remember that God Himself breathed His Spirit into me, and my job was to nourish that Spirit with the Word of God. So at work, I thought of these verses:

". . . so that the thoughts of many hearts will be revealed. And a sword will pierce your own soul too" (Luke 2:35).

Above all else, guard your heart, for everything you do flows from it (Proverbs 4:23).

During the time of my chemo sessions, because the therapy weakens the immune system, I did not attend church where many gathered. Instead, I meditated with much fervor and spent a lot of time in the Word of God. I especially focused on 1 and 2 Corinthians, of which Paul was the author. Paul, originally known as Saul, used to be an adversary of Christ. But God took His enemy and changed him. I used to think about the visions that Paul had about life and death. This gave me great encouragement. When my sickness was diagnosed, I bought a book, *The Complete Idiot's Guide to Breast Cancer* to learn more about cancer. The last chapter is entitled, "Facing Death Day to Day." Next to the title was a graphic of the grim reaper, dressed and hooded in a black robe with a scythe in his hands. I was scared to death of this graphic and refused to read that chapter.

Meditating on the book of Corinthians gave me something good to think about. I prayed that in the same way that Paul was able to carry the challenges of his life, I would be able to approach my challenges with the strength of the Holy Spirit. Paul also had a weakness in his flesh, and he asked God three times to remove it.

> *Three times I pleaded with the Lord to take it away from me. But he said to me, "My grace is sufficient for you, for my power is made perfect in weakness." Therefore I will boast all the more gladly about my weaknesses, so that Christ's power may rest on me. That is why, for Christ's sake, I delight in weaknesses, in insults, in hardships, in persecutions, in difficulties. For when I am weak, then I am strong (2 Corinthians 12:8–10).*

No other passage has strengthened me like this one; it gave me great relief from the guilt that resulted from my cancer. Instead of wondering why this happened to me, I started to proclaim the verse above. Rather than feeling guilt, I began to praise God for my weakness, from which I would gain my strength. What a great experience! Where I was once ashamed to admit that I had cancer, I now loved to let people know that I was a cancer survivor because that meant I got to proclaim that God was my strength. My thoughts were renewed; I could do everything through Christ Jesus who strengthened me. God gave me the boldness to take on more responsibilities that I had never taken before, and I began to experience and feel God's power flowing through me. Gradually, all my worries and fears about cancer began to disappear. How great is our God! When you ask God for the power, He will give it to you. I was privileged to receive this free gift. God in His mercy will not remember your past. All of my sins have been forgiven.

Today, I do not desire the life of comfort I once preferred. I have come to accept that life is a combination of health and sickness, comfort and difficulty, failure and success. When failure comes, rather than collapsing, it is important to think of failure as a step toward success. Through hardships and failures, we are made stronger.

In 2009, my husband and I had an opportunity to visit Jerusalem and Egypt. In Egypt, in the patio of our hotel room was a small palm plant, about one foot tall. It seemed to have been growing accidentally. Because I love palm trees, my husband tried to pull out the small plant so that we could take it back to America and plant it in our yard, but it did not yield. He thought that it would be easy to pull out such a small plant, but when he tried to pull it out he realized the strength of the small plant. I told him that the plant was growing in the desert. The plant is so strong because it has to grow deep roots to get its water. In the same way, when man walks through his desert, he has the opportunity to grow deep roots to get to his source of life, Jesus Christ, and to receive strength. God loved me so much that He allowed me to go through all of these struggles so He could resurrect me to be as strong as that little plant in the desert.

Do not think that you will be rejected by anyone because of your weaknesses or inabilities. No, in fact, God belongs to the weak. When we lay down our pride and confess our weaknesses to God, God will inspire us to great expectations.

Sunday is Coming

The mention of "cancer" immediately brings about thoughts of death, and it leads to a lot of fear. But there is no need to fear death; that is the message of Easter. Our life is meant to be lived without the fear of death. All those who live must die. The Bible teaches us that there are two types of death:

- The death that puts an end to our life possibilities
- And the death of our old man, which brings about rebirth

The second kind of death, the death of our old nature, gives us a chance to renew ourselves and to be transformed into someone new. To go through this type of death is a good experience because it creates a new heart within us, one without fear and with courage.

"Very truly I tell you, unless a kernel of wheat falls to the ground and dies, it remains only a single seed. But if it dies, it produces many seeds" (John 12:24).

The old nature is completely removed from us. Instead, the resurrected power now resides in us. We are moved from a dried-out state of mind to a lively new state of mind. Jesus said, *"The one who believes in me will live, even though they die; and whoever lives by believing in me will never die"* (John 11:25–26).

In Christ's life, Good Friday was the darkest of days. Yet, it did not stop Him from the resurrection. In my life, the diagnosis of my cancer, chemotherapy, and treatment was likened to Good Friday. It was the darkest of all days for me. Yet, I knew there would be a resurrection for me as well. I had already begun experiencing the power of the resurrection throughout my time of pruning. I saw the time of my trials as a temporary time of mourning and not as languishing. Before the resurrection, there was a Good Friday, but it is important not to get lost in that darkness. I believed that I was coming into a new season: new hair, new nails, new heart, and new thoughts. I was learning to appreciate the meaning of life and to turn my complaints into praises. Like a whirlwind that bends strong-rooted trees, life's struggles can bend you; nevertheless, you will eventually be realigned. God is my healer and I am cancer free. I was coming into a new season. I experienced a push from life that brought with it new power. I no longer felt like my old self. Instead, I felt like I could take on more responsibilities.

There was a song my mother used to sing in the mornings and the words sung out the truth of God's promises: no matter if life or death, I would have Christ with me. There was so much hope in that promise. The words of the song translate into something like this:

> With the resurrection power, we can receive
> eternal power. Whether I am living here on earth or
> living with Him in heaven, I am with Christ.

I began to have a changed mind. I no longer wanted to JUST live life. I wanted to live with purpose in everything I did. I wanted to take on more responsibilities. I no longer wanted to just sit back and let life take its course with me on the path. I wanted to be the one making the path. All my negative thoughts had vanished; instead, I knew that God was pushing me to do things with no limits.

From the west, people will fear the name of the Lord, and from the rising of the sun, they will revere his glory. For he will come like a pent-up flood that the breath of the Lord drives along (Isaiah 59:19).

All along, God wanted me to rise up and do more. I, unfortunately, had no understanding about the strength that lay within me. But when the breath of God came and breathed its life-giving spirit into me, the floodgates of my inner strength were opened, and I burst forth with an awakening.

In 1986 when my father died of cancer, I had a desire to help cancer patients, but that desire lay dormant. Seeing my father's agony and witnessing his pain brought such distress to my heart. I longed to help him somehow, and I believe it was from that source of distress that I found a longing to help other cancer patients. Unfortunately, it was just a strong desire in my heart that never went anywhere. I never actually did anything with that desire; I only sympathized greatly with cancer patients.

When David was anointed as a king he was only thirteen years old, but his reign did not take place until he was around thirty years old. God will finish what He has started, even if it is delayed. I read a story called *The Fern and the Bamboo* that uses great imagery to depict my thoughts exactly.

The Fern and the Bamboo[3]

One day I decided to quit . . . I quit my job, my relationship, my spirituality. I wanted to quit my life. I went to the woods to have one last talk with God.

"God," I said. "Can you give me one good reason not to quit?"

His answer surprised me.

"Look around," He said. "Do you see the fern and the bamboo?"

"Yes," I replied.

"When I planted the fern and the bamboo seeds, I took very good care of them. I gave them light. I gave them water. The fern quickly grew from the earth. Its brilliant green covered the floor. Yet nothing came from the bamboo seed. But I did not quit on the bamboo. In the second year, the fern grew more vibrant and plentiful. And again, nothing came from the bamboo seed. But I did not quit on the bamboo," He said.

[3] Turn Back to God Web site, "The Fern and the Bamboo," http://www.turnbacktogod.com/story-the-fern-and-the-bamboo/, Copyright © 2008–2012, turnbacktogod.com. All rights reserved.

"In the third year, there was still nothing from the bamboo seed. But I would not quit. In the fourth year, again, there was nothing from the bamboo seed. I would not quit," He said. "Then in the fifth year, a tiny sprout emerged from the earth. Compared to the fern it was seemingly small and insignificant. But just six months later, the bamboo rose to over 100 feet tall. It had spent the five years growing roots. Those roots made it strong and gave it what it needed to survive. I would not give any of my creation a challenge it could not handle."

He said to me. "Did you know, my child, that all this time you have been struggling, you have actually been growing roots. I would not quit on the bamboo. I will never quit on you. Don't compare yourself to others," He said. "The bamboo had a different purpose than the fern, yet they both make the forest beautiful."

"Your time will come," God said to me. "You will rise high!"

"How high should I rise?" I asked.

"How high will the bamboo rise?" He asked in return.

"As high as it can?" I questioned.

"Yes," He said. "Give me glory by rising as high as you can."

What God has started, He will finish. The battle is only in our minds. What I once believed I would never be able to do, God has changed my thinking to believe that I can do all things through Christ who strengthens me.

God has no use for the fearful. *"Anyone who trembles with fear may turn back and leave Mount Gilead."* So, *twenty-two thousand men left while ten thousand remained (Judges 7:3).*

Jehovah God chose Gideon to free the Israelites from the bondage of the Egyptians. But Gideon had hesitation because his clan was the weakest, and he was the least in his family. Gideon thought that his hope should rest on his status and his position, so he remained hopeless. But God assured him that victory would be given to the Israelites. Not sure whether or not this was a word that came truly from God, Gideon tested Jehovah. He prepared goat meat and bread, brought it along with the broth, and placed it on a rock that was shown to him by the angel of the Lord. The angel of the Lord touched the prepared meal and fire flamed from the rock, consuming the meat and the bread. It was then that Gideon realized that it was truly Jehovah God who was speaking to him.

God was with Gideon. A promise was given that no man would be able to defeat him. There were numerous soldiers along with Gideon, so a method was provided to find just the right kind of soldiers to accompany him. Those who were lacking courage and trembling with fear were free to go, and 22,000 soldiers left. Still, 10,000 were left. But God still thought there were too many soldiers. Again, they were tested. Out of a total of 32,000 soldiers, God selected 300 fearless men. With these brave soldiers, Jehovah freed the Israelites from the hands of the Midianites.

Strength is not found in numbers or in girth. It's not in denominations or in gender. It's found in a man's faith and in his trust in God's power. It's a belief that the power of God lies within us. It's that belief that allows people to do the will of God and to care for the needs of others with joy, not just to take on the needs of others, but to do it with joy.

Blessed is the one who perseveres under trial because, having stood the test, that person will receive the crown of life that the Lord has promised to those who love him (James 1:12).

As human beings, we desire the comfortable life. No one desires to carry a cross. But the Word of God teaches us that life brings failure, sickness, enmity, accusations, and hunger. Some people focus only on these negative things and quickly become depressed, but the Word of God also gives us strength to overcome all these things. We no longer have to be victims; we can become victors. That is the power of the Word of God. In testing, in sickness, or in experiencing a loved one's death we draw closer and closer to God.

We spend more and more time in prayer and meditation, and we receive strength from above. We should also think good and positive thoughts. Our thoughts should not control us; rather, we should control our thoughts. Like Paul, we should be able to take everything with joy.

We must transform our failures and sicknesses into opportunities. I decided to write this book, volunteer at a cancer center, and learn more about my area of expertise at work. Regarding work, I no longer wanted to do a so-so job. I wanted my work to be one of excellence. I wanted to be competent at what I did so that the reports I gave to the doctors were reports that exuded accuracy and quality.

When we go through sickness we receive the gift of patience. With our trust and faith in God, our fears will be removed. Our self-centered life will change; life will become purposeful and meaningful. Our talents and time will not be wasted. We will receive divine and holy thoughts.

From a young age, I never faced any kind of hardship. I always lived in comfort and so I always desired to continue to live in comfort. I never had the ability to truly understand the needs of others. Although I helped them with money and such, I did not have the capability to understand their anxieties. After going through my cancer, however, I learned to give thanks for everything. Thanks were on my lips with the very first opening of my eyelids in the morning. Thanks were in my breath with every meal I cooked. In everything I did, I gave thanks. My difficulties did not seem to be exhausting anymore; rather, they became challenges to overcome. Hardship is good. Pain is good. Those things will build character. Cancer (hardship) is a part of growth. Through prayer and meditation, you will persevere.

With this change of heart and change of mind, I left my old shell and stepped into a new resurrected life.

In the same way that Christ died and was buried deep into a cavernous tomb, our past life of hatred, jealousy, fear, anxiety, and lack of confidence must be buried. Again, in the same manner that Christ resurrected from the grave with power, we also must resurrect with power. We must be born again with new thoughts and a new mind that believes in the might of God.

Euroclydon, the Tempestuous Wind

I had passed through the hardest parts of my cancer. I had my breast removed, went through chemotherapy, and lost my hair. I found a great wig and my skin was renewed; I was brand new on the outside and on the inside. I reentered my world with this newfound life. Back at work, many of my co-workers noticed the change and they often commented on it. I even told my manager that I no longer wanted the light jobs. Instead, I wanted the more challenging jobs.

With this new outlook on life, I continued my day-to-day activities. My doctor prescribed 1 mg of Armidex as my preventative cancer medication and said that I would have to take it for five years. My life had become so routine that a co-worker commented that it seemed as if I had never gone through cancer at all.

My brothers, sister, and mother live in India. I was the one who called them frequently and spoke words of encouragement to them regarding my sickness. My cancer was diagnosed in June 2007, so that December, Christmas was celebrated with a deep gratitude in our hearts. We put up the tree, hung up the stockings, decorated our home, and gave multitudes of thanks to our God. To relay my joy, I picked up the phone to call my family in India, and when I spoke to my sister-in-law, Susan, I felt as if she was sad in her spirit and was keeping something from me. When I pushed her to open up, she refused. I knew something was wrong. She finally relented and told me that my older brother, Mathew, had found red swelling in his breast. Because he was well aware of my cancer, he went to the doctor to have the tumor biopsied. The day they received the results of the biopsy was the day that I had called. The tumor was found to be cancerous. I could not understand how this could be happening to two people in the same family. Was it not enough for one sibling to suffer with a dreaded disease? Why did my brother have to contend with cancer's grasp? I felt like a tempestuous wind had begun.

My family did not want to tell me the news of my brother because I had just started the recovery process from my own cancer. I had to explain and make them understand that I had no fear and that God had truly freed me from all heaviness and had given me a new life. So after convincing them of my changed heart, they gave me more details. I immediately told them that this was not the end, but only the beginning. *"This sickness will not end in death. No, it is for God's glory so that God's Son may be glorified through it"* *(John 11:4).* I quoted this verse to them to encourage them.

Even though I found words to give encouragement verbally, I felt heavy in my heart. To hear that there were two family members suffering through the same disease was hard to accept. Because he had just been diagnosed, I knew the anxieties and denial he would be facing. All of my family went through shock, pain, and agony . . . again. Two siblings had inherited a disease, one in India and one in America.

It is rare for males to contract breast cancer, so along with the depression of a disease, my brother faced embarrassment and guilt. The American Breast Cancer Society estimates that approximately 450 males die of breast cancer each year, and male breast cancer accounts for 1 percent of all breast cancer cases.

I lay on my bed and cried. I did not know what to do. I could not handle the news.

I decided to share the news with my children and my husband. My mind was soon wrapped up in pain. I went yet again to my closet and prayed, "Dear God, you once released me from my hopeless thoughts and anxieties. Please give that to my brother as well." I began to call him frequently, share my experiences with him, and share my hope with him, but he did not handle it well. He had to take pills to sleep at night. Finally, his doctor suggested surgery and chemotherapy.

He was taken to a reputable hospital, Lakeshore Hospital in Ernakulam, India, which provided advanced care similar to that given in the West. As Mathew was going through surgery and chemo, I was going through my recovery process. I would call him often and encourage him, but he found it difficult to endure the surgery and chemotherapy. He would tell me of his anxiety and that he could not sleep. He would often wonder why this disease was so prevalent in our family, and I would respond with the opposite. I told him that the disease was treatable and not life ending. I told him that God has chosen us to bring us to victory but that his job was to find the path to that victory. I told him that God is able to overcome all of these trials and that He wants to use our family to do greater things for His kingdom. Unless God pruned us, we would not be able to produce fruit. I explained that rather than looking at this disease from an angle of guilt, look at it from an angle of opportunity.

I encouraged him to continue to live life—garden, sweep the floor, walk—enjoy life, and continue to do what he did daily. I told him not to isolate himself to a room and look at himself as a disease-ridden person. When I explained the release that God had given to me and the freedom that God had brought to me, I could sense a bit of hope creep into my nearly seventy-year-old brother. I got him to see that we were a chosen people, not a despised people. God told us in 1 Thessalonians 5:14 to warn those who are unruly, comfort the fainthearted, uphold the weak, and be patient with all. Those are difficult commands to uphold unless you have the Holy Spirit of God inside of you. I got Mathew to see that God was working in our spirits by weakening our flesh so that He could sharpen our abilities to warn the unruly, truly comfort the fainthearted, uphold the weak, and be patient with all.

I told him that this sickness was temporary. It was just a matter of time before the disease would be removed. I told him that he would come into a new season and that God would open up the doors of heaven. I told him that the more obedient he became, the more blessings he would see.

My brother also went through the exact treatment I went through. He had a mastectomy done, went through six months of chemotherapy, lost his full head of hair, lost his appetite, had nausea, and finally was prescribed a preventative drug to continue for a period of time. Through it all, I had the opportunity to walk with him through his pain and anxieties. Even though we were thousands of miles apart in two separate countries, we were able to talk to one another through his disease. It's amazing that the first person I had a chance to counsel was my own blood.

As I told my brother of the counseling groups I attended and the volunteers who so kindly provided external things like makeup and wigs, my brother noted that India was very different from America. In India, all diseases are kept hidden. It is uncommon to talk about your sicknesses in public. Support groups are rare. So Mathew truly appreciated the help that I was able to give to him through my words; otherwise, he would have to suffer in silence.

Thank God that even though Mathew also had to endure the pain of cancer, the good Lord was with him and healed him from this disease.

BRCA2 Gene Mutations

When my son-in-law, Dr. Binu Philips, who is a physician, heard the news of my brother's cancer, he told me that my cancer might not be due to environmental causes but that it might be genetic. He recommended that I get tested to find out if the cancer was in fact genetic. When I went in for my routine checkup, I told my surgeon, Dr. Roshni Rao, about my brother's incident. She also recommended that I get tested to determine if the cancer was genetic. Although I had two professional recommendations, I was still scared to see the results. If the test came back positive, it would mean that both my daughters have a higher chance of contracting the disease. I was filled with guilt and despair. My daughter, Benji, must have sensed my hesitation because she kept pushing me to get tested. Because of her persistence, I got tested and found out that I had BRCA2 gene mutations. The National Cancer Institute describes it this way:

> In normal cells, BRCA1 and BRCA2 help ensure the stability of the cell's genetic material (DNA) and help prevent uncontrolled cell growth.

Mutation of these genes has been linked to the development of hereditary breast and ovarian cancer.

A woman's lifetime risk of developing breast and/or ovarian cancer is greatly increased if she inherits a harmful mutation in *BRCA1* or *BRCA2*. Such a woman has an increased risk of developing breast and/or ovarian cancer at an early age (before menopause) and often has multiple, close family members who have been diagnosed with these diseases. Harmful *BRCA1* mutations may also increase a woman's risk of developing cervical, uterine, pancreatic, and colon cancer. Harmful *BRCA2* mutations may additionally increase the risk of pancreatic cancer, stomach cancer, gallbladder and bile duct cancer, and melanoma.

Men with harmful *BRCA1* mutations also have an increased risk of breast cancer and, possibly, of pancreatic cancer, testicular cancer, and early-onset prostate cancer. However, male breast cancer, pancreatic cancer, and prostate cancer appear to be more strongly associated with *BRCA2* gene mutations.

According to estimates of lifetime risk, about 12.0 percent of women (120 out of 1,000) in the general population will develop breast cancer sometime during their lives compared with about 60 percent of women (600 out of 1,000) who have inherited a harmful mutation in *BRCA1* or *BRCA2*. In other words, a woman who has inherited a harmful mutation in *BRCA1* or *BRCA2* is about five times more likely to develop breast cancer than a woman who does not have such a mutation.[4]

Because I had such a high risk of recurring cancer, my doctor

_____

[4] "BRCA1 and BRCA2: Cancer Risk and Genetic Testing" *National Cancer Institute.* 2010 May 28. <http://www.cancer.gov/cancertopics/factsheet/Risk/BRCA>

asked me if I would like to have my other breast removed. I told her no. I asked her if there was any way to assure this cancer would not return. She said there was no way. I thought, *How many things exist in medical science that cannot be controlled by man!*

This news upset me so much. I cried knowing that I had passed this gene to my two daughters. I asked God not to use my sins or transgressions against my children. Even more daunting than experiencing my own cancer was the thought that my children might one day have to endure this disease. I hid the report and entered my prayer closet yet again, and I cried and prayed to my God. God removed my tears and brought me new hope and light with the following verse: *"I remain confident of this: I will see the goodness of the Lord in the land of the living. Wait for the Lord; be strong and take heart and wait for the Lord"* (Psalm 27:13–14). So I stopped worrying and started believing in the goodness of the Lord. I had to believe the goodness instead of worrying about the troubles of tomorrow, which are not in our control.

Soon after I received this promise, my older daughter, Susan, who had been married for seven years and remained childless, brought me the best news a mother could hear at the time. She was pregnant! This brought such a deep joy to my soul.

I decided to let the report say what it wanted. I was determined to live my remaining years with joy, peace, and responsibility. I would no longer worry if the cancer would return or if my children would get the cancer. I decided in my deepest of hearts to stop worrying, and I prayed that my children would also be free of these fears that lay in things they could not control. Instead, I prayed they would be given the best gift of all—to receive strength to take any challenge that comes their way. Soon, my youngest daughter, Benji, also came to me with some good news. She had passed the Bar and would be able to practice as a lawyer!

"Surely your goodness and love will follow me all the days of my life, and I will dwell in the house of the LORD forever" (Psalm 23:6).

My thinking has changed. I no longer expect an easy life; rather, I know I have an inner strength to handle all the difficulties that will be thrown my way. I know my burden will be light because

I do not carry it; God carries it for me.

"I only know that in every city the Holy Spirit warns me that prison and hardships are facing me. However, I consider my life worth nothing to me; my only aim is to finish the race and complete the task the Lord Jesus has given me—the task of testifying to the good news of God's grace" (Acts 20:23–24).

Paul's journey to Rome was filled with danger. They chose to listen to the owner of the ship and set sail even though Paul perceived differently and advised them not to. When the tempestuous winds hit, they thought they could fight the storm themselves. They took shelter around an island; they threw out everything that was heavy to make the ship lighter and even threw the ship's tackle overboard with their own hands. The Euroclydon was a cyclonic wind that blew through the northeast and had caused the ship Paul was traveling in to wreck. It was so devastating, and they had struggled for several days, bringing any hope for life down to nothing. But then, in the midst of their desperation, Paul received an encouraging word from the angel of the Lord. He was given a vision about their safety and told that he would escape because he had to stand before Caesar. This word of hope carried him and his men for fourteen days in the Euroclydon. They found hope in the midst of their tempestuous storms and found strength to continue to fight.

The way we react to the storm is what makes us or breaks us. We may think that we can fight the storms of life ourselves, but then we and fail miserably. In the same way that the Euroclydon darkened the light of the moon and stars, the storms in our life—death of a loved one, sickness, job loss—can cause us to lose faith and live in darkness. But don't give up, for it is during these times that we must immerse ourselves in prayer and meditation because prayer can remove all fear and anxiety from us. We must hold the hands of the One who has more power than the Euroclydon. In the midst of the storm, we must realize the value of the things around us. We must throw away the things that *seem* precious to us. When we relieve ourselves from the things that hold us back (pride, power, and prestige), our burdens will be lightened, and we will receive hope. We cannot escape the storm, but we should remain in the storm and feel the presence of God through it. The storms will make us much stronger and give us more power, more courage, and more faith. In other words, we will experience freedom from bondage. Through the storm, Elijah ascended into heaven. We will also ascend into the heavenly abode by the mighty hands of God Himself.

Since we live in a fallen world, we will always have storms; that is a reality. The type of storm for each one of us may be different. My storms were the news of my cancer and my brother's cancer, which occurred at the same time. There was also the news of my BRCA2 being positive, which meant I have a higher chance of the cancer recurring. But what could I do? No one could remove this storm from my life. If I tried to solve this on my own, I would have become more depressed and anxious. I learned, instead, to give my burden to God. These medical reports are no longer etched in my brain; I am stress free. I believe He will carry me to the end of my life without any fear of the sickness. I do not hope for a life without storms, but I believe He will hold my hand through it all. Why should I fear? The One who has control over all storms is with me. He has promised me that He will never leave me nor forsake me.

For every one of us, there will be a time when we have to face the storms of life. Each of us will experience our own unique challenge. During that time, we may lose hope and courage, and we will realize that we are not as strong as we thought. It is a time when the things we value most will become worthless or invalid. To endure these storms, we must be brave enough to throw out those things that weigh us down. For me, it was pride, self-sufficiency, selfishness, desire for comfort, and unbelief in God. Only when worldly pleasures are thrown away can life really be lived. In addition, those who have survived the monsoons of life have a responsibility to encourage and support others who will come to weather their own storms.

Arise, shine; for your light has come,
and the glory of the Lord rises upon you.
(Isaiah 60:1)

Although I was momentarily on the mountaintop and received a bit of hope and courage, I found myself going back into the valley of despair.

My brother's sickness, along with the results of the genetic tests, caused me to begin worrying about the future. Again, I started to lose hope. I began to understand the mentality of those who live without hope. Darkness started to settle in as negative thoughts plagued my mind. So I began to pray and as I prayed, I began to see that all the things I was worrying about were outside of my control. It was time for me to hand over these worries, over which I had no control, to the One who had ultimate control. I also realized that while I had no control over the span of my life, I did have a hand in the quality of my life. Regardless of the length of my life, I knew I wanted a life lived with quality. That quality comes from the work I put into it. I did not want to be a slave to the anxieties that came from worrying about my future. During my time of meditation, my Lord showed me a wonderful verse from His Word: *"Arise, shine, for your light has come, and the glory of the LORD rises upon you"* (Isaiah 60:1).

The verse was written in the present tense, so I knew that the glory of the Lord was already upon me. It's not that my light would come at some time in the future, but that it had already come. Darkness and sorrow may cloud the minds of unbelievers, but those who believe should not wallow in their misery. I was a believer. I knew that I was a child of Jesus Christ. I knew that I came from a royal bloodline. *"But you are a chosen people, a royal priesthood, a holy nation, God's special possession, that you may declare the praises of him who called you out of darkness into his wonderful light. Once you were not a people, but now you are the people of God; once you had not received mercy, but now you have received mercy"* (1 Peter 2:9–10).

So, rather than continuing life in the darkness that lurked around the corner, I felt a fire creep up inside of me that burned to proclaim loudly the freedom that God gave to me. I knew that it was important to stop watering the seed of worry. I knew I needed to cut off that branch and instead believe in the providence of God, accept the forgiveness of God, and live under the mercy and grace of God.

Then the angel said to them, "But the angel said to them, "Do not be afraid. I bring you good news that will cause great joy for all the people. Today in the town of David a Savior has been born to you; he is the Messiah, the Lord" (Luke 2:10–11).

Christ's birth replaces fear with courage, and sadness with joy. The good news of Christ says this: *"The Spirit of the SOVEREIGN LORD is on me, because the LORD has anointed me to proclaim good news to the poor. He has sent me to bind up the brokenhearted, to proclaim freedom for the captives and release from darkness for the prisoners, to proclaim the year of the LORD'S favor and the day of vengeance of our God, to comfort all who mourn"* (Isaiah 61:1–2).

When I read this verse, I realized that it wasn't just cancer patients who suffered from depression, but there were many who were slaves to this enemy. The Holy Spirit of God will free all those in bondage. Because God loves us so much, He gave His only Son to die on the cross and bear our burdens and to free us from slavery.

Life is full of challenges, and those who cannot handle the difficulties are usually the ones who fall into depression because hardships often come unexpectedly. But Christ teaches us that life comes with many hardships and when you accept that fact, you accept reality. The One who overcame all of life's burdens is with us, right here with us! When we believe that we do not have to face our struggles alone, but that Christ stands with us, then we can have faith to believe that we will have victory. To understand this fact, we need the Holy Spirit's blessing.

To the men who walked with Jesus Christ for three and a half years straight and experienced his miracles, He spoke about His future death and resurrection. When Peter heard about his Lord's horrible death, he could not accept it and in his denial he exclaimed, "No Lord! This will not happen to you!" It was impossible to accept the suffering of Jesus Christ and to imagine Him on the cross when Peter looked at it with human eyes. In fact, Jesus called Peter and said, *"Get behind me, Satan! You are a stumbling block to me; you do not have in mind the concerns of God, but merely human concerns" (Matthew 16:23).* There is such a huge lesson to learn here. Only with the Spirit of God can you take all of life with joy: failure and success, sickness and health, sorrow and joy. The Holy Spirit of God will gradually help His children step out of self-pity and find opportunity and purpose in the midst of their struggles.

It was Peter—who denied Christ because he could not handle the gut-wrenching stress of Christ's foretold death—who Christ went after and to whom He revealed His risen body. Christ had a love for Peter that was so great that even Peter's complete denial could not shake that love.

When Christ revealed himself to Peter after His resurrection, the Lord asked Peter three times whether he loved Him. The first time, Peter casually responded that he did love Him. But Christ pressed further, wanting Peter to gain insight. The second time, Peter said he loved Christ, but again his heart was seemingly distant. It was only on the third time that Jesus presented the question that Peter probably felt the guilt of his denial and understood the commission that Jesus was giving him. Indeed, in his third response, Peter finally said, with regret in his voice, *"LORD, you know all things; you know that I love you." (John 21:17).* Jesus asked Peter three times in this exchange whether he loved Jesus. Why was Jesus pursuing Peter? Peter had denied him three times and was lacking in his dedication to Christ, but still Jesus wanted to use Peter. Peter's past did not stop Jesus from carving out a future for him. Jesus knew what Peter was capable of, provided that Peter surrender all to Christ.

So, the Peter who was afraid of the reality of life was chosen by Jesus and given the Holy Spirit on the day of Pentecost, and by this gift, he began to live fearlessly. Only with this Holy Spirit did he begin to truly transform into the shepherd who would feed the flock. Do you see the transformation? The same worldly Peter who, before Christ's death, sought in his mere flesh to protect Jesus (from a divine appointment of suffering and shame) had been renewed into a man who learned to endure hardship with the Spirit of God. Listen to what he said after he had been transformed: *"Therefore, since Christ suffered in his body, arm yourselves also with the same attitude, because whoever suffers in the body is done with sin. ² As a result, they do not live the rest of their earthly lives for evil human desires, but rather for the will of God"* (1 Peter 4:1–2).

In the beginning, I questioned why cancer was devouring my family. Was it because of my sins or my parents' iniquities? I did not like the suffering, and I prayed that these kinds of things would not come upon our family. These worries grew into deep-rooted fear. But today, I have been transformed. Let my medical reports say what they will. I have the Spirit of God to accept all things! My prayer was, and is, that my daughters would receive this Spirit so they also can overcome the trials of life.

The worldly man has no desire to live life with all its hardships; he has no desire for sleepless nights or difficult situations of any kind. He only desires to live an easy life with no struggles. When challenges and failures come about, he quickly becomes depressed. But if that man seeks out the Holy Spirit, God will empower him to overcome life's struggles. As humans, we often depend on our own wisdom and abilities, but it's impossible to face difficult circumstances in our own strength. Desire instead for the Holy Spirit of God because He will give you the strength that you lack. God gives the Holy Spirit to all who ask, without any discrimination. *"Ask and it will be given to you; seek and you will find; knock and the door will be opened to you"* (Matthew 7:7). This a huge promise that is given to everyone who earnestly seeks. Your job is to find a desire within and be earnest in your asking. Rather than depending on men who are helpless, depend on God who is omnipotent.

The secret to a man's success lies in this verse: *"I can do everything through him who gives me strength" (Philippians 4:13)*. Those who hold onto God's promises can look at their failures and their struggles as a stepping-stone into another opportunity. Thomas Edison used to sell sweets on the train. One day a man, who didn't like what young Edison was doing, grabbed the boy's ears and threw him to the floor. This resulted in a life-long hearing disability for Edison, but Edison did not become overwhelmed with his injury; he went on in life to develop the phonograph, the motion picture camera, and the electric light bulb (among other things). I assume that his attitude was such that he saw his newfound weakness as an opportunity to keep from hearing undesirable talk.

Similarly, I once heard a fable about how birds formed their wings. This story teaches us that even our burdens are allowed/permitted by our Creator to enable us to fly:

> Birds were created without wings. Then God made wings and threw them out in front of the birds, and God told them, "Take these heavy wings and go!" The birds were able to sing beautiful melodies and grew stunning feathers, but they could not fly high into the sky. At first, the birds hesitated to take the newly created wings. But eventually, out of obedience, they did as God commanded. Using their beaks, they picked up the wings and placed them on their shoulders. Suddenly, the wings latched onto their bodies and they were able to soar through the sky. Even though the wings seemed heavy at first, their obedience allowed them to soar as if there was no load.

This story reveals a significant concept. Man can be compared to these birds that were created without wings. At times, God throws out in front of us a heavy load. We observe the matter carefully, but oftentimes we hesitate to carry the load because it seems too much of a burden. It is man's nature to shun responsibility, to turn away from troubles, and to remain apprehensive of such things. But if we make a decision to yield to God's discipline and bear our cross, the burdens that we once thought heavy will become light. The important thing is to do our part and yield. The birds obeyed despite their fears and put their wings on their shoulders, which then allowed them to soar! Our sicknesses and misfortunes will transform into opportunities when we surrender to God's direction.

When the children of Israel cried out to God, the Lord, in His compassion, sent Moses to deliver them from their slavery. In front of them was the Red Sea and behind them was Pharaoh's army. Bitter water was the only water available in Marah. Food was not available. The waters of the Jordan were floodwaters. But despite all of these huge obstacles, God would take them victoriously through it all. This is human life; we are slaves to many things, e.g., fear, hopelessness, inferiority, and guilt. These are not from God, but somehow we have come into bondage of these things. When we realize that these are not from God and cry out to Him, He will give us release. Before He gave the Israelites their release, He told them, *"On the first day remove the yeast from your houses" (Exodus 12:15).* We also have to remove all the yeast from our life; we have to remove the fears, guilt, and all that enslaves us. The Holy Spirit will help us to remove these things.

To see the land flowing with milk and honey, the Israelites had to go through difficulties. Without overcoming the obstacles in their lives, they could not get to the Promised Land. The great part of their journey was that God Himself showed up and removed their obstacles! He parted the waters of the Red Sea so that they became a wall on either side of them, He sweetened the bitter waters of Marah, He miraculously provided manna from heaven, and He provided water from a dry rock in the desert. Getting to the Promised Land is a journey filled with challenges, but God will be with us every step of the way. He will open doors for us and be our Provider.

The last obstacle that the Israelites had to face was the strong wall of Jericho. To bring it down, God instructed them to circle around it seven times and give a loud shout the last time around. Without questioning the logic of this strategy, they obeyed the voice of God; obedience and trust gave them victory. The Word of God is full of power. It even brings down strong walls.

The voice of the Lord strikes with flashes of lightning. The voice of the Lord shakes the desert; the Lord shakes the Desert of Kadesh. The voice of the Lord twists the oaks and strips the forests bare. And in his temple all cry, "Glory!" (Psalm 29:7–9).

In a Christian's walk in life, these types of walls exist—fear, anxiety, and hopelessness. The fear that is in front of us needs to be brought down; otherwise, it will cripple us. The fear of death will be far removed when our faith in God is built.

Even though the Israelites experienced all these miracles, when they arrived near the border of the Promised Land, they still hesitated to move forward because their fear of the land's inhabitants was greater than their trust in God. *"We saw the Nephilim there (the descendants of Anak come from the Nephilim). We seemed like grasshoppers in our own eyes, and we looked the same to them"* (Numbers 13:33). This is inferiority, to rely on our own strength and compare it to those around us instead of relying on God's strength and holding everything around us to His light. When we rely on ourselves, we may think of ourselves as grasshoppers. The Israelites actually wanted to turn back because of the inferiority they felt, but Joshua and Caleb stood up and said, *"Only do not rebel against the LORD. And do not be afraid of the people of the land, because we will swallow them up. Their protection is gone, but the LORD is with us. Do not be afraid of them"* (Numbers 14:9).

God specifically commands us not to fear man. When we remain ignorant of the Holy Spirit's strength in us and are unaware of the God-given breath that blows from our nostrils, we remain fearful and apprehensive. We look at most situations with anxiety and think that a task cannot be accomplished because we rely on our own strength. If we can instead see the power that lies within us, we will not look at ourselves as grasshoppers; rather, we will see ourselves as Holy Spirit warriors! The problem is on the inside. Remember, God has created us in His own image. What is on our inside is what is seen on the outside. If we think that we are slow or cowardly, then that's what will show on the outside. Instead, if we see ourselves as strong, courageous men and women who walk with the Holy Spirit of God, then that's what will show on the outside. It was the Israelites themselves—not others—who said they were like grasshoppers. It is important to practice this. We should compliment ourselves and convince ourselves that all things can be accomplished because we have God's own Spirit inside of us. Speak out loud that as long as God is with you, you are strong and you are capable. Speak it and say it so that your thinking begins to change. When I wake up at four thirty in the morning, the first thing I do is give thanks to God. Then, I tell myself that I can do all things through Christ who strengthens me. I spend time meditating on all the promises that God gave to me, I call to memory all the things that I have accomplished in my life, and I praise God for those things. So when I get to work, I do not think of myself as a cancer patient or that I am weaker than others. You must retrain your mind to think this way.

Once my thinking changed, I stopped having an inferiority complex about my disease. My co-workers even say from time to time that I am an inspiration to them. Psalm 139:14 says, *"I praise you because I am fearfully and wonderfully made; your works are wonderful, I know that full well."* Thinking of yourself as a grasshopper and seeing yourself as inferior actually blocks you from receiving the blessing of God. My cancer has been removed. I have no reason to think that I am a cancer patient. I realize that God has softened my heart of stone and given me renewed thoughts and a renewed mind. *"I will give you a new heart and put a new spirit in you; I will remove from you your heart of stone and give you a heart of flesh. And I will put my Spirit in you and move you to follow my decrees and be careful to keep my laws" (Ezekiel 36:26–27).*

Where I used to feel like God was punishing me through cancer, today I feel like God loves me, and allowed me to endure the pain of cancer so that I might have this chance to experience His mighty ways.

"Why do you now cry aloud—have you no king? Has your ruler perished, that pain seizes you like that of a woman in labor?" (Micah 4:9). God has given me thoughts of the divine. I have no enmity with others. I have a God-given ability to forgive. I used to be overly sensitive. Now, if anyone tries to provoke me, I no longer let the situation upset me; rather, I pray for them. It takes more control to forgive than to take revenge. I feel like I am doubly blessed and have an incredible

sovereignty inside of me. *"I will put my Spirit in you and you will live, and I will settle you in your own land. Then you will know that I the LORD have spoken, and I have done it, declares the LORD"* (Ezekiel 37:14).

When will your light shine forth like the morning?

1. When you share your bread with the hungry
2. When you provide shelter for the poor
3. When you don't hide yourself from your own flesh

When we do these things, then our light will shine out like the morning and our healing shall spring onward speedily.

Investments are necessary for living a financially secure life. However, most people invest in their temporary life here on earth. The average life span is only about seventy or eighty years. Eternity is much longer than that. So how do we invest in eternity?

Matthew 25 speaks of the divisions that will be made on Judgment Day. He will separate the lambs from the goats. To the lambs, he will offer the inheritance of heaven because they represent those who fed the hungry (both spiritually and physically), clothed the naked, and took in the stranger. He will cast the goats into eternal fire because they represent those who did the opposite by not feeding the hungry, clothing the naked, or taking in the stranger.

While we are alive, if we invest in others, we invest in eternity. We do not have to be afraid of judgment. We can live without fear. Although the news of my cancer should bring tears, it does not. I do not live in fear. I do not bathe in self-pity. Instead, I live with joy wanting to offer more to the world and do as much as I can for others. I also want to bring this joy to others who are also struggling.

The words of God had always been in my heart, but they were asleep. It was only through my struggle that they were awakened. The promises were gathered in one place, bound by floodgates. But when the gates were opened, the promises rushed forth in a fury. I became zealous for the Word of God.

"As for me, this is my covenant with them," says the Lord. "My Spirit, who is on you, will not depart from you, and my words that I have put

*in your mouth will always be on your lips, on the lips of your children and on
the lips of their descendants—from this time on and forever," says the Lord
(Isaiah 59:21).*

Rather than allowing the BRCA2 report to bother me, I held
on to this promise that what He had relieved me from would also
be passed on to the next generation and the next and the next. The
chains had been loosed. The promise was not just for me, it was
for my descendants! Through my misery, I received a call—ARISE
AND SHINE! And I did.

Because of unbelief, the carnal man becomes hopeless
when failures occur. When we meditate on the Word of God,
however, it will transform our unbelief and provide hope in the
midst of our hopelessness. It will renew the thoughts in the bottom
of our hearts and bring about what is now commonly referred to
as positive thinking. The thoughts that reside in the depths of our
hearts determine our successes or failures. Because the Word of
God is filled with treasure, meditate only on it and find the power
that rises within; it will move you. We have two choices: stay in a
depressed state of mind or arise and shine.

Let the weakling say, "I am strong!"
(Joel 3:10)

The book of Joel teaches us that God gives the Holy Spirit to ALL, not just to pastors, teachers, and priests. Whoever calls upon the Lord will receive the Holy Spirit and will receive hope. They also stand free of the final judgment of God.

After my surgery and my chemo treatment, when I reentered the world, I had a slight hesitation about being viewed as "different." How would it be to work with, travel with, and exist with healthy people when I only had one breast, was wearing fake hair, and was now seen as a cancer patient? I saw myself as a member of a different group, the cancer survivor group, the group that was now the weaker part of society. Even though I no longer had the disease, I would be labeled as the weaker part of society, as a cancer survivor. I had doubts as to whether I would be able to function in my everyday life like I used to. But despite these thoughts, I had a deep desire to overcome, and not just endure, my weaknesses. I wanted to rise up despite my limitations, and God strengthened me with Joel 3:10 and Zechariah 4:6:

Joel 3:10—Let the weakling say, "I am strong!"

Zechariah 4:6— "Not by might nor by power, but by my Spirit," says the Lord Almighty.

The awesome task facing Zechariah was to rebuild the temple, an undertaking that was both difficult and discouraging. There was opposition, both on the inside and the outside. The task seemed impossible in the natural. No one cared about the work, there were not enough materials, and there was so much to be done but not enough help to get it done. The message given in Zechariah, however, was that of faith: *"Not by might nor by power, but by my Spirit."*

In my life, I was my own opposition. It came from within. Even though we overcome our fears, it is very important to have a transformed mind, one that moves us from negative thoughts to positive ones. Matthew 12:45 says, *"Then it goes and takes with it seven other spirits more wicked than itself, and they go in and live there. And the final condition of that person is worse than the first. That is how it will be with this wicked generation."* This was part of a story that Jesus told about a demon that went about in dry places looking for a place to rest. Because he could find no place, he decided to go back to his original home and dwell there. The house was in clean condition, but no one lived there; it was empty. So the demon went and called seven other demons and took up residence in the empty home. In the same manner, even if you kick out one demon (like fear), if your heart remains empty, the displaced demon will come back with seven others even stronger than himself. Where there is negativity, fear will reenter. I had cast out the fear of cancer through all of my stages, but I did not replace that spirit of fear with the Spirit of God; I only cast out the fear. Thus, I remained empty and that's why I began to have doubt again. That's why I reentertained the thoughts of guilt and shame, because I was still empty. So in the mornings, after giving thanks to God, I always fill my head with positive thoughts. I encourage myself to believe that I can do all things through Christ. I recite all of these positive verses before I step foot into the world. My husband and I have regular prayer every morning, but even before that, I make sure and recite these verses out loud.

Even in my career, I started to believe that I would be more competent than before and that I would provide quality work. I was successful in replacing my fears with courage and reliance on God. Before I stepped foot into the front doors of the hospital, I prayed for the doctors, all the employees, and all the patients in the hospital. I also asked that God would not allow anyone to suffer because of my lazy work and that He would give me a good work ethic. God granted me my requests. I also desired to grow intellectually at work. I began to take initiative in reading more and attending more workshops about my area of work, microbiology.

God gave me a vision of my own talents and when they were revealed, I felt as if all these years I had dug them into the ground. Today, I do not like to see people live with negative thoughts. With all my might, I would like to help people become victorious, and I hope desperately that they will see the secrets that have been revealed to me.

What I went through was devastating and I hoped that no one would have to endure what I had to endure. Yet, God brought me to greener pastures, and He gave me rest. I know that I have to testify to this miracle in my life, but even for that, I have no words. So I asked God to provide a way for me to express my experiences into words, and He provided.

I loved being in my comfort zone and had no desire to get out of it. But God saw that there were talents hidden deep within and He had to push me out of my comfort zone so that I could discover my talents. Because of this push, I now have eyes to see the pain that others may have to bear and eyes to see the talents that lie within me. My selfishness had been replaced with selflessness. I began to realize that if I was going to be helping others then I had to be released from my bondage of fear, guilt, and depression; otherwise, they would not get any benefit. *They promise them freedom, while they themselves are slaves of depravity—for "people are slaves to whatever has mastered them" (2 Peter 2:19).*

I never prayed for the actual healing of my cancer, but the thing I greatly desired in my heart was to be freed from slavery. Even when I go and volunteer with cancer patients, I pray in my mind that they would be freed from their bondage of fear and hopelessness and that they would be given a new vision like God had given me. I want them to feel that it is not the end, rather only the beginning of their journey.

Persevering under trials is a strength that is given from God. To become a leader, you need perseverance. Jesus did not have to endure the cross because of any wrong done on His part. He also had to take the criticisms and accusations of many, but He persevered. In this world, to take leadership, we need perseverance. *"Blessed is the one who perseveres under trial because, having stood the test, that person will receive the crown of life that the Lord has promised to those who love him" (James 1:12).* Hang on during your times of trial and in the end, you will receive a crown. When we take adversity into our own hands we become easily discouraged, which can lead to disappointment and depression.

I realized that I could not take the pain of cancer myself. I told God about my helplessness and knew that no one else in this world could help me with the pain either. I handed over my pains to the One who is able to help, and the Holy Spirit strengthened me. It was through my sickness that God helped me to understand things I could not before. My unstable mind began to change. My narrow mind began to change. The sickness threatened me at the beginning. Now, I was the one threatening the sickness. Now, I am fifty-nine years old, and I believe that I can continue learning and that God will enable me to take on more responsibilities. This sickness is no longer an obstacle for me.

When we are young and healthy, strong and successful, we think we can do anything; we do not think about life's uncertainties, about life's struggles. With that type of mindset, when a great challenge occurs in our lives, our strength quickly flees. At that time, we realize that those whom we put our trust in (family and friends) cannot help us—not that they do not have a desire to help, but they do not know how to help—and that which we relied on (money and position) is of no use to us either. Even those who are close to us have their own struggles with fear, so how can they be of assistance to our own needs? When I was presented with my challenge, with the sickness of cancer, I was in a state of fear. But I quickly realized that I could not depend on anyone or anything around me. In addition, if I allowed myself to remain in fear, it would become contagious—my fear could make their lives miserable and filled with fear also. It was then that I realized that I needed to strengthen them also in the midst of my own struggles. So I began to meditate on God only. Through meditation, I was freed from pride and dependency on others. I was transformed through meditation into a submissive servant of God. God renewed within me that which I had lost—strength of mind. I told God that I was tired and felt rejected by my community. I knew that even though my family would help for some time, they also would get tired. So I asked God to give me strength to fight the battles in my head.

I went to Him with complete helplessness and believed so strongly that I would somehow receive more than all that I had lost. I never uttered a word of my despair to another human being, not even to my own husband. I did not want to share my anxieties with my husband because I loved him and did not want him to be burdened. My God showed me mercy. Without remembering any of my past, He gave me capacity and might. Although I would lose my strength every now and then, I had the Holy Spirit who went with me through that dark tunnel of my life. God did not give us a spirit of fear, but a sound mind.

I, the woman who used to see the difficulties in all situations, could now only see opportunities. *"For you were once darkness, but now you are light in the Lord. Live as children of light"* (Ephesians 5:8). I recognized that I used to walk in darkness. I should not only live for me, my husband, and my children. It is my joy now to exclaim out loud the love that my Jesus had for me and the mercy He will show to those who live in darkness, depression, loneliness, fear, and life-threatening sicknesses. At the volunteer center, when I see joy in the faces of the depressed and courage in the faces of the fearful, I become fulfilled in a way that I have never experienced before in my life. Just like Paul said in Corinthians, I too will boast all the more about my weaknesses so that Christ's power may rest on me. Today, I proclaim with pride that I am a breast cancer survivor. I am not a victim; I am a victor. I am the chosen one. What a privilege.

Today, when I look back at all these wonderful gifts that God gave to me, I end up in tears because I cannot understand why such a Holy God would give me so much of His Spirit. Why did God give me freedom from my slavery? My heart overflows with gratitude.

Those of you who may be reading this and feeling the way I used to feel, take heart! God has release for you as well. He rescued such a sinful lady as myself, and He will certainly rescue you as well. When the Holy Spirit is given to you, you with proclaim your strength.

"And afterward, I will pour out my Spirit on all people. Your sons and daughters will prophesy, your old men will dream dreams, your young men will see visions" (Joel 2:28).

When I was filled with this Holy Spirit, I woke up from my weariness and was ready to face my cancer. I told myself that I was strong enough to fight this cancer. Why? Because God was, and is, with me. Then I told myself I am strong, as it is proclaimed in Joel 3:10.

Both blessings and curses can be spoken by the same tongue. Whatever you proclaim will be carried out in your life. Perhaps the degrading words that we heard while growing up still haunt us, but to get release from that inhabitation, we must proclaim to ourselves victory, healing, and renewal. Our words and attitudes are the echoes that guide our actions.

What will you do in the thicket of the Jordan?

Of all the prophets in the Bible, I believe Jeremiah is the most heroic. He had to stand firm in the midst of persecution, disbelief, and ridicule. He had to minister to a decaying nation who refused to listen to anything he said. Despite his lack of influence, God enabled him to persist for forty years so that he could witness to a corrupt nation.

When Jeremiah was first called by God, he responded with his limitations saying that he was a young boy who did not know how to speak. But God encouraged him and said He would be with him. *"I have put my words in your mouth" (Jeremiah 1:9).* God chose him.

It was no easy ride. In fact, Jeremiah went through many hardships. On one occasion, because the officials did not like him, Jeremiah was put inside of a deep cistern (well) that contained no water, only mud. All prophets and leaders have to endure this kind of rigor. Joseph was first put into a pit and then into prison before he became Pharaoh's right-hand man. David was a mere shepherd boy who had to fight among lions and bears before he reigned as king on a throne. Although Moses grew up in the Pharaoh's palace and had all the privileges that his fellow Israelites did not have, he chose to abandon his place of authority to take his place amongst his brethren. It was after he left the riches of his forty years of palace life, when he was in the desert place, that he experienced God through the burning bush.

Paul never prayed that his troubles would be removed; instead, knowing that the future would hold many more trials, he

97

just trusted God and believed that God would set him free from all harm. In Acts 28, Paul had just arrived safely on shore from a tempestuous storm when he was bitten by a snake. With no fear in his mind, he simply shook off the snake into the fire he was building and continued. Those who witnessed this miracle believed he was a god.

It was the Holy Spirit that enabled these men—Jeremiah, David, Moses, and Paul—to persevere. When I meditated on the power these men were given, I became strong myself. I stopped desiring the easy life. I accepted that life was full of trials, but if I sought out the Holy Spirit, I would experience God through my trials.

My surgeon, Dr. Rao, told me that I am at high risk for having the cancer recur. The cancer, she said, could come back in my brain, liver, spinal cord, and such. And yet, for some, the cancer would never come back. According to my genetic tests, the risk of reoccurrence is high. But that risk is neither in my control nor in the control of the doctors. One thing I do believe is that the God who could deliver me from the cancer is with me.

"When your words came, I ate them; they were my joy and my heart's delight, for I bear your name, LORD God Almighty" (Jeremiah 15:16).

Man always strives to be on top. Some desire to become leaders, but each level of success comes with its own share of struggles. God never promised us a rose garden without thorns. In fact, God has said that life will come with tribulation, but that does not mean we must abandon joy. In fact, as we enable the Holy Spirit to subdue our torments, we release within ourselves an unstoppable joy. So, anticipate troubles and hardships in life but receive the Holy Spirit of God and you will become equipped.

Dead Sea Experience

$\mathcal{A}$fter my surgery, chemotherapy, and recovery, I had a chance to visit the Holy Land in Israel. Before I flew out there, I was very excited about the idea of visiting the Dead Sea, the Garden of Gethsemane where Jesus prayed, and Marah, the location where water was miraculously provided to the Israelites during their wilderness experience. WOW! To think that I, in my short lifetime, would be able to experience firsthand the locations that Jesus walked was an absolute thrill. Before leaving, I excitedly bought clothes to wear in the Dead Sea. Although I did not know how to swim, I was ready to swim in this salty water, which allows you to float without any effort of your own. The Dead Sea is one of the world's saltiest bodies of water; it is 8.6 times more salty than the ocean. The salinity makes it impossible for animals to thrive. It has been known to carry a high density of minerals and cosmetics have been made from its extraction.

When I finally experienced this long-awaited and eagerly expected trip to the Dead Sea, the tour guide warned us of the dangers of the salt; we were told not to allow the water to get into our eyes and not to lie in the water longer than fifteen minutes. Our tour group decided to separate the men and the women so that each group went into the water together. A lady I had befriended on the tour and I entered the water together. I lay on my back and let the current float me. With my head held up to prevent water from entering my ears, I lay there with my eyes shut not wanting to let the water enter my eyes. I assumed that the lady who had entered with me was laying there beside me. Only later did I find out that she had decided at the last minute that she did not want to wade in the sea and had actually left my side. Although she told me she would float with me, she became afraid of the water and left at the last minute, without giving me any warning. I had no idea I was floating alone.

There was a sign at a distance into the sea that warned people not to go beyond that point.

After floating for some time, when my body started tiring, I opened my eyes to see who was around me. To my fear and shock, I was alone. No one was anywhere around me. The depth of the water where I entered was only knee deep, but when I tried to put my foot down in the water I was lying in, my foot did not reach ground. I knew I had floated out to the deep. I started to become a little afraid. I prayed in my fear and remembered my husband; my husband has a heart of gold and would go the ends of the earth to protect me. At that moment, my Lord blessed me with a most appropriate Word from Isaiah 43:2: *"When you pass through the waters, I will be with you; and when you pass through the rivers, they will not sweep over you."* So even though I had no friend and no husband there with me, I had the Lord there with me. I began to repeat this verse over and over so that I believed it with the innermost part of my soul; I did not want to believe the thoughts of fear. Pretty soon, my fears were gone, and I received hope and strength. I believed that, even though I was alone in the Dead Sea, had been separated from the rest of the group, and did not know how to swim, I would be rescued. I believed because meditating on the verse enabled me to believe. When I opened my eyes and looked above me, I saw a walkway with steps close by. I moved closer to the steps, but due to my inexperience with water, I could not turn my body and place my foot on the step. To my surprise, I saw a man walking on the walkway above. I called out to him and asked if he could help me. He reached down, grabbed my hands, and tried his best to pull me out of the water, but try as he might, he could not lift my weight on his own. Not knowing English, he babbled something to me in Arabic and left. I was alone yet again in the waters of the Dead Sea with no friend and no husband. My body was quickly tiring, and I began to feel anxious. So the Lord strengthened me yet again with another Word: *"For he will command his angels concerning you to guard you in all your ways" (Psalm 91:11).* I realized then that the man who had passed by could not pull me out on his own. Right then, I saw two men walking by on the walkway! I knew God had sent them to rescue me; they were like two angels to me. I called out to the two men asking for help. The two of them held each one of my hands in their own hands and was able to lift me just enough to land my feet on the steps that led to the walkway. They did their deed and went on their way. I climbed out of the water and walked back to the tour site. Two men who I had never seen were prepared by my Lord to be my angels during my time of need. How trustworthy is the Word of God! Since then, I have such an incredible faith in the power of God's Word. Even in the Dead Sea, God rescued me! He did not allow my husband or my friends to rescue me; He prepared two strangers to rescue me.

I learned a huge lesson from this incident. John 10:12 says, *"The hired hand is not the shepherd who owns the sheep. So when he sees the wolf coming, he abandons the sheep and runs away. Then the wolf attacks the flock and scatters it."* The lady, my friend, who had entered the Dead Sea with me left me alone, not because she was evil, but because she herself was fearful of the sea. We often rely on those who are afraid themselves and in the end, we become disappointed because they cannot rescue us. But the truth is that in all of life's experiences we must look upward to Jesus; He is the only One who can rescue us. Man cannot fulfill that role; even those who say they will be there to help you might not be able to fulfill their promises to you because of their own limitations.

Jonah, a prophet in the Bible, ran away from God and got on a boat to sail to Tarshish. But God sent a strong wind to make the waters, on which Jonah was sailing, violent. He was in the midst of a huge crisis, but the Bible says that during this extremely turbulent time, his eyes were on God above. Jonah's prayers were received and God indeed rescued him. Deliverance comes from God and God alone, so our eyes should always be focused up above, not on those around us.

During my Dead Sea experience, when I tried to place my feet on the ground and found that I was no longer in shallow water, I became scared. It was when I looked upwards that I saw the two young men who were able to help me.

The Bible describes Job as a man who was blameless and upright. But even this man had to endure extreme trials. He lost all of his possessions, his children, his wealth, his health, and suffered with disease. His friends came by to comfort him, but none of them were able to do so. Job says of them, *"I have heard many things like these; you are miserable comforters, all of you!" (Job 16:2).* He longed desperately for the days of his past when his joy was full. In his suffering, Job questioned God's justice. He saw himself as a righteous person. *"If I have walked with falsehood or my foot has hurried after deceit—let God weigh me in honest scales and he will know that I am blameless" (Job 31:5–6).* Job could not understand why he had to suffer. In the end, God finally argued His omnipotence and asked Job some questions that stilled his thoughts. Job, realizing how small he was in the midst of all of God's creation, replied, *"I am unworthy—how can I reply to you? I put my hand over my mouth. I spoke once, but I have no answer—twice, but I will say no more" (Job 40:4–5).* We see God when we see our unworthiness. Finally, in chapter 42 of the book of Job, we see Job's testimony. He puts his trust back in God, acknowledges that God can do all things, and that nothing He wants to do can be thwarted. After seeing God and after his trust was restored, he confessed, admitting that he questioned God because of his limited understanding. He admitted that he had only heard about God before, but now after *seeing* God, he despised himself and repented in dust and ashes (Job 42:6). That was an overwhelming repentance. This is the victory of submissive faith.

After his confession, he prayed for his friends and God ended up blessing him with twice as much as he had before. When we read and hear about God, our understanding is limited. But when crisis comes, if we allow God to speak to us and we allow ourselves to experience Him, we will come out of the crisis with twice as much as we had before. When we come upon trouble in our lives, we yearn for God's presence to give us peace.

When I learned about my sickness, I questioned God and asked why I had to endure this. What had I done wrong in my life that I had to bear this great disease? I became angry. In the end, I confessed to God the greatest sin in my life: I had no faith in

God. Though I grew up a Christian, married a Christian, and went to church regularly, my understanding of God was horribly narrow. I had no idea of the extent of God's might and His omnipotence. I was able to look within and see where my weakness lay— in my faith. Like Job, I also repented greatly for my lack of faith.

When I was diagnosed with cancer, and prior to my surgery, some of the ladies in my community who had also gone through cancer themselves came to pray for my anxiousness and for my fears. They came to encourage me. Much later after my surgery and treatment, when they saw me at a church convention, they saw me as a different person, with a pleasant face. One of the ladies commented, "Oh! You are like Job. It seems that God has given you twice as much in your soul than you had before your surgery." After my sickness, I experienced more strength, confidence, and hope than I had before my sickness, and she was able to read that in my face.

One day I was outside gardening with my two-year-old granddaughter, Abriana. A neighborhood dog barked and she barked back. It seemed that she had no fear of the big dog. A few minutes later, when she had a little distance from me, the dog barked again. This time, instead of barking back, she ran to my side. When she was close to me, she had no fear. When she was far from me, fear settled in. This is how life is.

Big dogs (like cancer) will bark at us, but if we are walking with God, we can bark back rather than cower in fear. When crisis comes, rather than drowning in self-pity, we should spend more time in prayer and meditation so that the severity of the crisis can be seen as slight in comparison to the omnipotence of God. Meditation really helped me to see how powerful God was. My meditation times were spent repeating the Word of God over and over to myself. I cried with an insatiable craving for God's presence. It was during those times of meditation that I received faith and strength. Through His mercy, He sent His words and strengthened me, healed me, and delivered me from the weakness in my mind.

The Sea of Galilee and the Dead Sea can be compared to two types of characteristics in man. The Sea of Galilee both receives and gives water daily, which causes life to flourish. The water is clear and full of fish. There is an abundance of life. The Dead Sea only receives water but does not give, so it is dead. No life can exist in its realm, much less flourish. Likewise, some men, although alive, are dead. In selfishness, they have nothing to give. All men will die, but the Word of God will live forever. Our labor of love to those less fortunate will never come back void. No, those acts of kindness will be multiplied back to us a thousand times over.

Jubilee Year

Leviticus chapter 25 tells us that when the Israelites arrived in the Promised Land, God told Moses to honor the Sabbath. They were told to cultivate the land for six years and the seventh year was to be celebrated and kept aside as holy. No one was to harvest in the seventh year; rather, they were to pick freely from the fields and give it to the foreigner and to the servant. The seventh year was to be set aside seven times every seven years for a total of forty-nine years. In the fiftieth year, a trumpet was to be sounded and the year was to be celebrated. It was a jubilee and was to be consecrated, set aside as holy. Freedom was to be proclaimed.

This was a huge celebration for the Israelites. All debts were canceled and everyone had a chance to start over. All prisoners were set free. It was a time of freedom. What a joyous time it must have been for the Israelites. They were given grace! They were given liberty.

This is how the fifty-sixth year of my life could be described. I was given a death sentence, but after realizing what a powerful God I served and after repenting for my lack of faith, I heard the trumpet sound! I believed that God intended a special purpose for me—that I had been consecrated. I was given freedom from my guilt, shame, anger, and fear. My cancer year was my year of jubilee; it was a time to celebrate. The negative thoughts that kept me a prisoner for so long had been refashioned into thoughts of praise. Rather than continue life with a downcast face, I was able to face not only my cancer with boldness but every other thing that would be thrown my way in the future. My broken heart was finally healed, and 2007 was a year of favor from the Lord. Even though I first asked, "Why me?" I realize now that it was really just the preface to the favor that was waiting to be rendered to me. All of my debts had been canceled, free of charge! I felt like a lottery winner.

My thoughts transformed into jubilee thoughts. Discouragement turned into joy. Sickness turned into health. I began to see things differently. I began to expect God's favor over and over. I wished that I had these kinds of thoughts during my youth.

In order to enter into this type of liberation, you must first have repentance. I *was* focusing on my past sins, those that I committed with and without my knowledge. But I developed a conviction, which led to an insatiable hunger for God's presence. I began to believe that I would be liberated, freely and without any effort of my own. This can be described as faith.

The next requirement for liberation is forgiveness. We receive forgiveness from God freely; now it's our turn to forgive freely. When God so freely gave me His forgiveness, an expectation had emerged—I was to offer that type of forgiveness to others. Not only that, but I had to receive forgiveness for myself.

To experience redemption's fruit, we have to forgive others without any reservation. So I decided that I wanted that power, the power to overcome my own anger, my own emotion, and replace it with forgiveness. I did not just want to forgive someone who had physically hurt me; I also wanted to be able to forgive those who made petty, but insulting or irksome comments as well. Today, I have the strength to overlook people's negative comments, whether spoken purposefully or not. I just remind myself that they may be having a tough day and their negative remark may be a result of their stress. Oftentimes, I end up praying for them. My forgiveness is not a benefit to the other person; it's a blessing for myself, because when I forgive, I do not harbor feelings of anger, which lead to stress. I remain calm and peaceful. What a powerful prayer Jesus Christ taught us while He suffered on the cross: *"Father, forgive them, for they do not know what they are doing" (Luke 23:34).*

Why Should We Forgive Others?

First of all, accept that we need forgiveness. When we receive that forgiveness, we are blessed. Unfortunately, many times, we desire greatly to be forgiven by God, yet we do not extend forgiveness to others. To be able to forgive requires an inner power, which comes from God.

Jesus illustrated the concept of forgiveness in the parable of the unmerciful servant in Matthew 18:21–35. A king who wanted to settle accounts with his servant ordered the servant and his family to be sold as compensation for the servant's large, unpaid debt. The servant pleaded for his life, and the king took pity and canceled his debt. However, this servant later came across his peer, who owed the servant a smaller debt. The unmerciful servant began to choke the debtor and ordered immediate repayment. He ignored the debtor's cries for mercy. The servant finally had the man thrown in jail. When the king found out about his servant's unmerciful actions, he was furious and had the servant tortured until he paid back all that was owed.

The servant's behavior is very typical, even today. We get forgiveness from our King, but we do not offer forgiveness to others. Since I received forgiveness from my Lord, if I do not offer forgiveness back to my peer, I will also be treated as the servant in the story. I do not want that anger from the Lord.

God's Unconditional Love

Jesus loves us without any conditions. Luke 15:11–31 tells the story of the prodigal son who went and squandered all his father's wealth and finally returned back to him when he came to his senses. The father held no grudges and welcomed him back with open arms. Verse 17 says, *"When he came to his senses, he said, 'How many of my father's hired men have food to spare, and here I am starving to death!'"* The prodigal received enlightenment. We need this type of illumination; we need to come to our senses.

When the prodigal son went back to his father's house, there was a great celebration to honor his return. The same was true of my return to God. After I had left His home and spent all that I had, I finally came to my senses. When I had been illuminated with the truth of God, I went back to His house, He received me with open arms, and there was great rejoicing because another soul had been saved! All my debts had been canceled. I had been set free; it was a time of freedom. My jubilee had arrived.

> *The Spirit of the Sovereign LORD is on me, because the LORD has anointed me to preach good news to the poor. He has sent me to bind up the brokenhearted, to proclaim freedom for the captives and release from darkness for the prisoners, to proclaim the year of the LORD's favor and the day of vengeance of our God, to comfort all who mourn, and provide for those who grieve in Zion—to bestow on them a crown of beauty instead of ashes, the oil of gladness instead of mourning, and a garment of praise instead of a spirit of despair. They will be called oaks of righteousness, a planting of the LORD for the display of his splendor. (Isaiah 61:1–3).*

Verse 1 says the Spirit of God is in me. It does not say that it will be in me in the future; rather, it is here now, in the present. When the Spirit of God comes upon a man, all thoughts of depression, anger, fear, and sicknesses are released. This favor is already with me because the Spirit of God is already in me. There is health with my name on it. For worldly people it may seem impossible, but with jubilee comes health, happiness, fearlessness, strength, etc. God can do anything.

I am a jubilee-minded person now.

In the same way that our body needs food, our Spirit needs the Word of God. The Word of God is what enables us through any and all of life's circumstances. Crisis only brings us closer to God. In prayer, I become closer to God. With meditation, I receive more strength.

Only One Chance at Life

We will never be able to return to our past. The footprints we have made cannot be erased. I decided that sharing is very important. It is important to share time, money, skills, and knowledge. The experiences we have with God need to be shared. This is what has encouraged me to write this book, so that I can share my experience with you.

We should not live only for ourselves. As Jesus states, when we give to others and share what is ours (whether that be material or immaterial), we will have done it for Jesus as much as we have done it for the person in need.

> *For I was hungry and you gave me something to eat, I was thirsty and you gave me something to drink, I was a stranger and you invited me in, I needed clothes and you clothed me, I was sick and you looked after me, I was in prison and you came to visit me. Then the righteous will answer him, "Lord, when did we see you hungry and feed you, or thirsty and give you something to drink? When did we see you a stranger and invite you in, or needing clothes and clothe you? When did we see you sick or in prison and go to visit you?" The King will reply, "Truly I tell you, whatever you did for one of the least of these brothers and sisters of mine, you did for me" (Matthew 25:35–40).*

God set me in a good position in life; He created me and put me into a good family setting, gave me a good education, gave me a comfortable life, and put me into Christian surroundings. But because of my own laziness and selfishness, I chose not to use the talents that were obvious to me and also was not aware of some of the gifts that God had placed in me.

When my sickness was diagnosed, it was a big shock to me. Cancer meant that my days were numbered. I no longer had a long life ahead of me. Life was too short. Many years had already passed and many years were still to come. When you consider life, man's average life span is about seventy or eighty years. In the grand scheme of things, seven or eight decades is nothing; it is too short. Therefore, this life should be lived with great responsibility not only toward ourselves but toward our community. I should give my all to serve my people, my nation, my country, and my world.

Moses experienced the constant and good provision of God, and he remembered that life was short. Psalm 90 relays his prayer of remembrance. Verse 12 says, *"Teach us to number our days, that we may gain a heart of wisdom."* This is an extremely important verse. When I was notified of my cancer, it was as if someone took a large hammer and pounded me on the head and finally woke up my sleeping brain to think "LIFE IS SHORT." Realizing that our days are numbered gives us wisdom. Rather than wasting the rest of my short life, I felt as if I *had* to take on more responsibility. I felt as if I *could* take on more responsibility, and I felt that God *would* enable me to carry the load.

Luke 13:6–9 says, *"Then he told this parable: 'A man had a fig tree, growing in his vineyard, and he went to look for fruit on it, but did not find any. So he said to the man who took care of the vineyard, "For three years now I've been coming to look for fruit on this fig tree and haven't found any. Cut it down! Why should it use up the soil?" "Sir," the man replied, "leave it alone for one more year, and I'll dig around it and fertilize it. If it bears fruit next year, fine! If not, then cut it down."'"*

It is not common to find a fig tree in a vineyard. Thinking that the tree would bear good fruit, the owner planted the fig tree, but when it was time for the harvest, no fruit was found. Disappointed, the owner told the keeper of the vineyard to cut down the tree. That which does not bear fruit is useless and it only steals space and nutrients from those around it. In the same way, I felt that I had not bore any fruit my entire life. I felt that I had just existed and was taking up space only. Even though God planted me in the middle of a thriving vineyard, I myself did not thrive. God gave me the best opportunities but I wasted it. I felt like I needed to make up for all the years that I had used up carelessly.

The realization of my wasteful life developed an insatiable desire to change, to become more responsible in life, to shoulder a greater burden for others, and to accomplish more feats. I wanted to be the best in every area of my life. I wanted to be a hard worker, a more competent employee, a great mom, a bold mouthpiece for sharing God's Word, and an excellent wife. I no longer wanted to live with mediocrity. I wanted instead to soar on the wings of eagles and fly!

During the time of my surgery and chemotherapy, I could not help but be in awe of the sacrifice that my doctors endured so that they could serve me in their best capacity. I wondered how many years of their life were spent studying and working to gain the expanse of knowledge they had within. Because they sacrificed their sleep, their pleasures, their own well-being, I was given the best treatment possible.

When our heart is ripened to desire good things, things that will benefit others, God opens doors! Everything we want to do at that time becomes possible. Nothing is impossible when your state of mind is in the middle of God's will. The thing that I absolutely could not handle during my time of sickness was not the physical pain, but rather the pain in my mind. When God had finally given me victory and when my thoughts had become jubilee thoughts, I empathized deeply with those who were suffering the same way that I had been suffering. I intensely wanted to share my revelation with others. At first, I did not think I could do so; I did not think this book could be written, but God enabled it because it was His will to provide this type of revelation to His people. I believe that I have an amazing future ahead of me. I believe that God is elevating me, that He is drawing me up from a deep pit and pulling me up to much higher ground.

Although I began my journey thinking that my sickness was the end of me, I realize today that it was just the beginning. Who would ever think that Abraham's wife, Sarah, after she became menopausal, could bear a child? What man thinks is impossible is possible with God.

Rather than just focusing on my distress and pitying myself, I saw a vision of myself rising up and being able to help others. *"I remain confident of this: I will see the goodness of the Lord in the land of the living"* (Psalm 27:13). The soil of my heart was fertilized with hope. The depression in my mind had vanished. I no longer saw myself as a sick, cancer patient. I now saw myself as a renewed, empowered warrior of God who had been given a call in life to bring good news to the brokenhearted, to set captives free, and to release the oppressed. I had decided to get out of my comfort zone. I began to have visions of greatness; I began seeing myself excel. I began to realize who God had created me to be. I had finally been given sight; the blinders had been removed.

When I began to use the small talents that I knew I had, God placed His powerful hand over mine and enabled me to do much more than I anticipated. I have accomplished so many more good things in life after my cancer than I had ever done prior.

In 2007, at fifty-six, I finally heard the trumpet call. "You are released." My debts were canceled and replaced with abundance. Discouragement had turned into joy. Sickness was turned into health. It was my year of jubilee.

All men desire freedom; no one wants to be a slave. Unfortunately, those who claim to walk in freedom are chained to things like fear, guilt, and shame; for these people, nothing in life will bring joy—not advancement in position, education, or wealth. Furthermore, no person can free them from their chains. They can only be released through the Word of God. Only His mercy can unchain them from the unfavorable and, instead, bring thoughts of jubilee.

A New Brand

"Therefore, if anyone is in Christ, the new creation has come: The old has gone, the new is here!" (2 Corinthians 5:17).

Every day before work starts, we have stand-up meetings where we are free to talk about anything we would like. Typically, a supervisor or senior technician leads these meetings. One day, the manager asked one of my co-workers to lead it. Immediately, another co-worker commented, "She is too shy." The manager quickly responded, "No, she is not too shy; she is reserved."

In life, we are given many labels by friends, family, co-workers, and even by strangers at times. We are branded as shy, outgoing, friendly, demanding, austere, sweet, etc. Even parents name their children with a label. *Jabez was more honorable than his brothers. His mother had named him Jabez, saying, "I gave birth to him in pain" (1 Chronicles 4:9).*

Sometimes we even label ourselves, and most of the time the labels we hear about ourselves are negative. Sooner or later, we begin to identify with the negative labels we are given. We believe we are shy or demanding or austere.

Just like the spies who saw themselves as grasshoppers when compared to the giants in Canaan (Numbers 13), we may see ourselves unable to handle the great obstacles before us. This is usually a result of trusting in our own strength rather than relying on God's Holy Spirit. Of course, we cannot handle it on our own because we are weak in our own abilities. We are only strengthened when the Holy Spirit of God comes upon us.

One day, I went to visit my daughter's friend, a thirty-one-year-old who had been in the hospital after having surgery to remove a benign uterine tumor. She had just fallen asleep prior to my visit due to the pain medication she was taking. I waited there talking to the girl's mother. When she finally woke up, she told me she wanted to show me something. She took out her cell phone and showed me a picture of the tumor that used to live in her uterus. This was a reminder to me of the way most people are. Rather than letting go of things in our past, we tend to hold on to it. Our past may include both good and bad circumstances, but the past is the past. It is over. All that is waiting is the future. Second Corinthians 5:17 tells us that those who are in Christ are new creations; the old has passed, and the new is yet to come. What a great promise this is. God does not remember our past, no matter how bad it was. Whether we were raised in a horrible family, abused by the ones who were around us, or physically defeated by sickness, God will give us a new name if we believe. This new label can only be attained through faith.

Joshua chapter 2 describes the story of a woman who was redeemed despite her sinful past. Rahab was a prostitute who followed pagan gods. But when she heard of the wonders that the Israelites' God, Yahweh, had performed in the desert and through the Red Sea, she began to develop a faith in their God. Through this bit of faith, she helped the Israelite spies and made them swear to save her and her family. Because of her faith, not only was her entire family was saved from annihilation, but she was transcribed into the genealogy of Christ! It did not matter that she was a prostitute. God rescued her because of her faith! Because of Rahab's faith, her family was also delivered: *"But Joshua spared Rahab the prostitute, with her family and all who belonged to her, because she hid the men Joshua had sent as spies to Jericho—and she lives among the Israelites to this day"* (Joshua 6:25).

Similarly, 1 Samuel 16 recounts the story of David, a mere shepherd boy who was elevated to the position of king. After God dethroned King Saul because of Saul's disobedience, the Lord instructed Samuel to go to Bethlehem in search of the new king.

God specifically told Samuel not to focus on outward appearances. So Samuel, the prophet, arrived in Bethlehem and immediately went to sacrifice to the Lord, as God had commanded. Along the way, he saw Jesse and invited him and his sons to the sacrifice. *"When they arrived, Samuel saw Eliab and thought, 'Surely the LORD's anointed stands here before the LORD'"* (*1 Samuel 16:6*). But God told him not to look at his appearance or height, so he asked Jesse to present his other sons. Jesse presented seven of his sons before Samuel, but God told him that none of them were His chosen. Samuel finally asked Jesse if he had any other sons, to which Jesse replied, *"There is still the youngest,"* Jesse answered. *"He is tending the sheep"* (*1 Samuel 16:11*). When Jesse's youngest son, David, finally arrived, God acknowledged him to be the chosen one.

The father of David, Jesse, obviously did not consider his youngest son to be anointed of the Lord, perhaps because he was just a shepherd boy or because he was the youngest. But the good Lord looks at our heart, not at our outward appearances. He does not look at our status in life, our careers, our experiences, or our past; He just looks at our heart.

These passages brought such encouragement to me. God does not hold our past sins against us, nor is He limited by our weaknesses.

I tested positive for the BRCA2 gene, which is essentially a mutated gene. This means my daughters are at high risk of getting cancer. In fact, I can even have a recurrence of cancer. My surgeon asked me if I wanted to remove my other breast as well. But I believe with all my heart that God can remove this mutation, or He will provide the strength that is needed for me and my daughters to handle the sickness if it were to come.

Some people may think that this hereditary gene is a form of a curse, passed down through the generations. But I believe that God can remove this curse. I believe that all of our past sins have been forgiven. I cried to God for my family. Just like Rahab, I also cried out to God, and I believe that our healing and our deliverance has already been written. During my times of prayer, I believe that I already have received. I do not think that I am waiting to receive it, but that it has already been handed down to me. Mark 11:24 says, *"Therefore I tell you, whatever you ask for in prayer, believe that you have received it, and it will be yours."* I believe with all my heart that the deliverance that was given to the prostitute, the forgiveness that was bestowed, and the freedom that was realized has also been given to me.

My prayers for my children, my family, and for other cancer patients are the same: that God would give the Holy Spirit to them as well. There is nothing that I can offer, but the Holy Spirit of God is given freely to those who desire Him, and there is nothing more precious, more valuable, or more useful than the Holy Spirit. The best gift that we can give to our generation is prayer, especially prayer that the Holy Spirit would dwell within them.

In 2 Kings, after they had crossed the Jordan River, Elijah said to Elisha, *"Tell me, what can I do for you before I am taken from you?" "Let me inherit a double portion of your spirit," Elisha replied. (2 Kings 2:9)*

Mahatma Gandhi, in his autobiography, said that we save money and possessions for our children because we do not have confidence in their abilities. Rather than worrying about our children, just pray for them and trust that God will give them wisdom, knowledge, and will clear their paths so that they can make good decisions in life. Believe that God will give them the strength to face any challenges that life may throw their way.

When I applied for my American citizenship, I was asked whether I wanted to change my name. Although I did not change my actual name, my identity has changed since I became a true believer of Jesus Christ. I no longer feel the same, make decisions the same way, talk the same, or even look the same. My character is more patient and more prayerful than it was before I knew God.

In Genesis 17, God changed Abram's name to Abraham. *"No longer will you be called Abram; your name will be Abraham, for I have made you a father of many nations. I will make you very fruitful; I will make nations of you, and kings will come from you. I will establish my covenant as an everlasting covenant between me and you and your descendants after you for the generations to come, to be your God and the God of your descendants after you. The whole land of Canaan, where you are now an alien, I will give as an everlasting possession to you and your descendants after you; and I will be their God" (Genesis 17:5–9).*

116

God Himself changed Abram's name and elevated him to a much higher position than the one to which he had been born.

Paul of Tarsus, whose Hebrew name was Saul, was *"of the people of Israel, of the tribe of Benjamin, a Hebrew of Hebrews; in regard to the law, a Pharisee" (Philippians 3:5)*. After the conversion, he described himself as a servant of Christ Jesus, called to be an apostle, set apart for the gospel of God. While talking to the masses, he described his position in life as a zealot for the law to the point of killing Christians. After his conversion, he described himself as a slave to Christ. Paul endured a lot of difficulties for Christ—he was beaten, he was trapped in storms, he was put in jail—but the Bible says that even when a snake came and bit his hand, he simply shook it off as if it was no big deal. He believed that God was his protector and that God would enable him through his trials. Paul said in Acts 14:22: *"We must go through many hardships to enter the kingdom of God."*

In 1 Corinthians 15:55, he bravely asked, *"Where, O death, is your sting?"* During my time of chemotherapy, while I was all alone, I meditated on this verse in silence. I began to believe that I lived with God and I would die with God. Those who are fearful cannot be used by men, nor by God. No one wants to suffer in life, including me. It is easy to give up the fight when you are suffering, and it is difficult to fight the hardship. Most people will give up when trials become too intense. But those who walk with the Holy Spirit of God do not give up; they stay and fight. They see it as a temporary trial and look forward to the great things that lie ahead. During my time of chemotherapy, I was looking ahead to my exciting new future, not focusing so much on the difficulties of the chemo. I knew in my mind that the time of suffering would quickly be behind me.

Winston Churchill stated, "Optimists see opportunity in every danger, the pessimist sees danger in every opportunity." I want to be an optimist. Since 1986, when my father was going through cancer, I wanted to help cancer patients, but I never actually did anything about it. When I personally went through the pain that came with cancer, I began to have a much deeper understanding of the needs of a cancer patient. When I was an observer of the disease back in 1986, I wanted to give money, but now as a survivor who has endured the distress, I know that there is much more to give. I saw my disease as an opportunity to take action on my desire. Thus, I write this book to help others.

"A man is but the product of his thoughts. What he thinks, he becomes. Your beliefs become your thoughts, your thoughts become your words, your words become your actions, your actions become your habits, your habits become your value, your value becomes your destiny."—Gandhi

Going through this sickness allowed me to discover my weaknesses and my strengths. I felt like I had wasted my talents and my time. Because I did not want to come out of my comfort zone, I remained a caterpillar who could not transform into the butterfly. But God pushed me out of my comfort zone so that I could form wings and fly. A caterpillar was never meant to stay a caterpillar. By crawling into its version of a tomb (a cocoon) and dying to its former life, a caterpillar can be completely transformed into a different creature altogether, a spectacular butterfly. This metamorphosis brings about a totally different lifestyle for the once earthbound caterpillar. With new capacities of flight, the butterfly gets to enjoy a far superior realm of reality than in its former life as a weed-eating worm with legs.[5]

According to what Paul says in Romans 7:20, man tends to do what he does not want to do because of indwelling sin. When sin grows, it leads to anxiety, depression, and hopelessness; it tends to bring about laziness as well. As a cancer patient, I experienced these depressive feelings. No one likes to be at this stage—where you feel bound to your depression. I desired greatly to be freed. I knew I did not want to be under the control of these negative thoughts and when I prayed to be released, what I received was a steadfast mind. This was my transformation, my metamorphosis. The old thoughts had been thrown away. Just like a caterpillar grows beautiful wings and flies to its newfound freedom, I had grown beautiful wings and was flying free. No doctor, friend, or person can bring about this freedom. Only the Holy Spirit can provide this kind of freedom. This is what it means to be born again.

---

[5] Story taken from http://www.rocktribe.org/metamorphosis.html

How Can You Be Born Again?

First, you have to realize that you are under the control of sin. Second, you need to develop a desire to be free from sin. Third, you need to believe that only Christ can give you this freedom. You must go to the Person who can give release and ask Him for it. Romans 8:1 says that when we receive this freedom, our burdens are made light so that we can face whatever problems may come our way. To sense the weightlessness in an overburdened heart is incredible! There is a long-lasting joy in this type of heart. When this kind of heart was given to me, I could not help but gleefully think that I was the owner of such a joyful heart.

Matthew 17 describes a time when Peter, James, and John went up to a mountaintop with Jesus and saw Jesus transfigured with a great light beaming from within. Then, they saw Jesus speaking with Moses and Elijah. What a terrifying yet amazing time this must have been for these disciples. They probably never wanted to leave that place or that feeling. This is how we are often. We do not want to come down from the mountaintop; we want to remain in the place of glory. But God wants us to come down because there is work to do, and there are hardships that need to be boldly endured as a warrior of Christ. Immediately after their mountaintop experience, as they were going back down, they came across a boy who was plagued with epilepsy. Although the disciples tried, they could not heal the boy. Jesus Himself had to heal him. When they asked Jesus why they could not drive out that demon, He replied, "Because you have so little faith." These disciples had just come down from a divine experience with God, but they lacked faith!

For fifty-six years of life, I stayed within my comfort zone. But in my fifty-sixth year, God pushed me out of my comfort zone because He saw the potential within me. Through my sickness, I feel like He has anointed me with His Spirit to welcome the discomforts. I can relate to the psalmist in Psalm 92:10: *"You have exalted my horn like that of a wild ox; fine oils have been poured upon me."*

Some people, when given responsibility, feel burdened with the chore, but those who are concerned about others take the responsibility with joy. It actually brings satisfaction to their soul.

Like the verse above in Psalm 92 says, in order to take the burden of others, fine oils have to be poured on you; in other words, you must be empowered by the Holy Spirit.

Be bold to repent because God removes you from sin's entanglement. Sin is inherent in man, but unrepentant sin will bring guilt and unhappiness; it will lead us to feel that our lives have been wasted. So remove yourself from the grasp of sin. Rather than looking at your past failures and distance from God, run toward what lies ahead—the opportunity for renewal. A renewed mind transforms you into a new man, so clothe yourself with the new man.

Seasons of Life

There is a time for everything, and a season for every activity under the heavens:

> *a time to be born and a time to die,*
> *a time to plant and a time to uproot,*
> *a time to kill and a time to heal,*
> *a time to tear down and a time to build,*
> *a time to weep and a time to laugh,*
> *a time to mourn and a time to dance,*
> *a time to scatter stones and a time to gather them,*
> *a time to embrace and a time to refrain from embracing,*
> *a time to search and a time to give up,*
> *a time to keep and a time to throw away,*
> *a time to tear and a time to mend,*
> *a time to be silent and a time to speak,*
> *a time to love and a time to hate,*
> *a time for war and a time for peace.*

(Ecclesiastes 3:1–8)

Solomon was a man to whom much wisdom was given, and in the verses above, he reminds us about the seasons of life. There is value to analyzing these different seasons; they are similar to the seasons in nature—winter, spring, summer, and fall.

Winter

Everyone prepares for winter. It gets cold and so it is necessary to prepare for this season. Likewise, we must also prepare for our trials. We must draw close to God during this time, and He will draw near to us. This season is somewhat lonely also—people do not go out as much. But everyone has to face winter. During this time, people will isolate themselves from others to stay away from the cold. This is winter. But winter does not last long. It eventually dissipates into spring. In the same way, our sicknesses and trials are just for a season. Spring will come soon. Some think that winter will never leave—there is no hope for the next season—but we must dream for the new season. Our trials are temporary, and we must wait quietly for the salvation of the Lord. Our personal winters teach us valuable lessons in life: patience, gratitude, humility, and love. We learn all of these things during the cold and lonely seasons of our life; it is a time of training.

Spring

Spring is a beautiful time of year. We see flowers blooming, rain falling, and trees blossoming. When a man has gone through his winter and fall and enters into spring, his face will shine. New fruit will grow. But in order for this to happen, we must stick through the winter by continuing to hope that a new season will arrive. During our spring season, we will be continuously producing fruit. Because our old skin was shed during our fall season, we have newness in spring. New beginnings. New thoughts. New responsibilities. This newfound strength and outlook in life does not come from within; it comes from God. When we survive winter, our fears will be removed. We will be given courage to move forward to the new seasons.

Summer

Summer is the season of play, vacations, and enjoyment. People go on cruises, kids play outdoors, families grill, and people go to pool parties. Summer is a time for delight. The seeds that we sowed in winter can be reaped in summer. We must give thanks for our winters, for the hardships in life. Because we went through the dry and cold season, we will receive positive changes.

"The life of man is like the seasons of the year, each with its peculiar beauty. Whatever be the season, choose the life that is noblest, for custom can make it sweet to thee—" (Hobart Huson, author of *Pythagoron*.)

Autumn/Fall

Autumn or fall is a season when the trees lose their leaves— they fall off. In the same way that the old leaves fall off, during our autumn season, our old man is shed away. Everything that is bad should be shed. Things that will break relationships, harm communities, and promote laziness should be thrown away. We will receive a renewed might to strengthen others, help our community, take on the burden of others, and be generous with our resources and time.

Therefore, if anyone is in Christ, the new creation has come: The old has gone, the new is here! (2 Corinthians 5:17).

Just as there are seasons—winter, spring, summer, fall—for the weather and surroundings, there are seasons to our lives. There are good seasons and bad seasons, but the important thing is to move forward and not get stuck in one season. Some people always want it to be spring; they do not want to endure the harsh winter season. But God's Word teaches us that life presents both spring and winter. When this thinking becomes a reality in our lives, we become enabled to weather the storms of life rather than engaging in self-pity. In addition, most of us do not prefer change; we would rather have one season for all our lives. For me, the change was good. It helped me to adapt to a new situation, and it allowed me to grow on the inside. The most important thing I learned through my difficulty was to dismiss the negative talk that I sometimes heard around me, and especially the ones that were directed toward me. Whereas I used to get aggravated by negative remarks made toward me, I now have been given perspective to see such remarks from another angle. I understand that some people may be having a bad day or maybe something happened in their past that caused them to think or speak a certain way toward me. Rather than becoming angry at those who speak negatively, I have been given grace to forgive them and pray for them.

I feel so blessed to be relieved from the stress and anxiety that can come from harboring anger. I wish I had this kind of spirit when I was young. I realize that God wanted me to grow from the rigidity in my head, so He gave me a new mind. He has brought me to my season of growth.

Season of Growth

Pruning is the method of cutting off the unfruitful branches of a plant or tree, removing all the unproductive parts of a plant so that nutrients can be redistributed. The time of my cancer was my time of pruning. I was more than willing to cut off the unfruitful cancerous part of my body. Of course, the surgery and chemo were painful, but my fear of cancer pushed me to endure this pain. I went through a mastectomy (removal of the breast), which was not only physically painful but also mentally agonizing. I was afraid to look at the breast that had the cancerous tumor in it, so the idea of removing it brought a sense of relief. In fact, I told my surgeon, Dr. Rao, to rush and remove it because I did not want it to spread. I also endured the nausea and effects of the poison that was injected into me through chemo. Human doctors pruned my body, but the Word of God pruned my soul. John 15:1 says, *"I am the true vine, and my Father is the gardener."*

Because God pruned me, I received hope. Jeremiah 29:11 says, *"For I know the plans I have for you,' declares the LORD, 'plans to prosper you and not to harm you, plans to give you hope and a future.'"* God had a plan for my life. The best part of my pruning process was receiving a MOST PEFERCT verse at the RIGHT MOMENT to strengthen me; I knew God was with me through every step of the process.

"For the word of God is alive and active. Sharper than any double-edged sword, it penetrates even to dividing soul and spirit, joints and marrow; it judges the thoughts and attitudes of the heart" (Hebrews 4:12).

Even though I had read the Bible during my youth, it had never become alive for me. During my time of pruning, the Word of

God was very present, and it offered so much truth in my life that it transformed my dead faith. I began to believe with all my heart and knew in the deepest parts of my soul that what God was saying was true. Faith had now been instilled in me. Today, I pray that God would not remove that faith from me. I know that I will need that faith for the rest of my life.

I experienced more strength during my time of pruning. I believed that if I could endure the trials of cancer, I could endure anything in life. After my surgery, I spoke with one of my cousins who is a bishop of a church. I told him that I wished I had some tough times during my childhood. The bishop responded by saying that perhaps God saved this type of trial for this time in my life because He knew that I would not be able to endure this kind of difficulty during my youth. God knows the right time to prune. These kinds of trials will bring us to a place of deep, revelatory faith, and that faith will empower our minds. This mental power is a FREE gift from God. It is given to all who desire; God does not look at our background to discern who should or should not be given this gift. He simply gives to all who desire. A successful life requires a strong mind, and this mental power is greater than physical strength.

Learning to Fly

When a baby eagle is around forty-five days old and about forty times their birth weight, its mother will cause a great commotion in the nest so that one of the babies gets scared and falls out. The baby, at that point, does not know how to use its feathers, and it will fall and flap around with great fear. Right in the nick of time, the mother eagle will catch the baby and fly it back to its safe nest. This process is repeated until the baby eagle learns to fly.

We are often like the baby eagle, wanting to rest in the safety of the nest. When troubles come, we wonder if God has abandoned us, but during our free fall, right before we hit the ground, God comes to our rescue. My cry to God is like the cry of the psalmist:

"Answer me when I call to you, my righteous God. Give me relief from my distress; have mercy on me and hear my prayer" (Psalm 4:1).

I thank God that He has enlarged me in my distress and that He has given me new determination. Rather than swim in self-pity, God has enabled me to walk on the firm ground of newfound faith. He has given me a broad vision, new ideas, and new thoughts. I believe that I really *can* do all things through Christ.

Our successes, health, and wealth will not last forever. Neither will our sicknesses or failures. In times of riches, learn to live with humility and be good stewards of your resources. In times of misfortune, look eagerly toward hope and learn to cultivate purpose.

The Real Enemy Within

"Without knowing what I am and why I am here, life is impossible."—Leo Tolstoy

God called Moses to lead the Israelites out of slavery. He was saved from death as a baby when other baby boys were being killed, and he grew up in the house of Pharaoh, the very person who was trying to kill his kindred. He grew up with the opulence, education, and training that could only be attained by growing up in the Pharaoh's house. But when God called Moses, he replied saying that he was not an eloquent speaker. Although he was given everything in abundance up to this point in his life, all that Moses could focus on during his time of calling was his weakness. Despite his inability to see God's provision thus far, God provided a mouthpiece for him in Aaron, his brother.

So together, Aaron and his brother Moses went to speak to Pharaoh. Aaron remained with Moses until Moses had built up the courage to go on his own. The point is that God provided! When Moses felt incapable, God provided a helpmate. Sometimes, God will give us people to help us overcome our difficulties, and other times God Himself will show up in the form of the Holy Spirit. Either way, God is the Provider. It is important to move on from the point of fear, and not remain in a place of hesitation. Just like Moses was eventually able to approach Pharaoh on his own, without Aaron, we too must persist to take the steps on our own, without "Aarons" to help us.

I read a story that helps to clarify this thought. One day while an old man and his wife were driving to their destination, the man stopped the car to purchase some cigarettes. He stopped the engine, left his wife in the passenger seat, and walked up to the cigarette store. As he was walking, he noticed that the car was parked at a slant near a huge ditch, and it had slowly started to roll toward the ditch with his wife inside. He cried out to his wife to stop the car and in desperation, quickly ran to push the back fender to try to stop the descent, but the car was too heavy and ended up rolling over him and killing him in the process. Because the brakes malfunctioned, the situation had gotten out of control. Our human brain works like the car; when it malfunctions, we end up in uncontrollable situations. Malfunctions of the mind occur when we allow things like bitterness, unforgiveness, and anger to take root. To keep the mind functioning properly, we must maintain it daily. Daily. Not every once in a while, but daily we must forgive and pray for those who hurt us and seek the strength of God. God created us in the power of His own strength. We were born with the breath of God inside of us. When we live life without nourishing this gift from God, we fly out of control and lack faith. As a result, we suffer things like depression, incapability, fear, etc. This is the enemy within, and we all know what our enemies are. We must take the initiative to fight it. We must yearn to figure out the truth, because as the saying goes, the truth will set you free (John 8:32).

The life we are given is very short, so if we remain a slave to the enemies within, we will not be able to enjoy our lives. It is important to acknowledge our accomplishments in life—whether large or small. Just like God, after His creation of the world, said, "It is good," we, too, must learn to find beauty and contentment in the works of our hands.

When my husband and I bought the house we live in now, I had no idea about houses, how to decorate them, or what to do in the designing of a house. Without any prior knowledge, I helped choose the brick color, the wall paper, the colors inside, the carpet, etc. Once the house was built, everything looked beautiful. Many of my friends who came to visit complimented us on how beautiful the house was. I did not even know that I had this talent in me.

After my cancer, I remembered all these things and realized that I have a lot of talent within, but oftentimes I failed to use my talents. Negative thoughts would keep me from being productive. After my healing of cancer and after the healing of my mind, these thoughts were transformed, and I began to accomplish so much more. The more I did, the happier I became. Instead of thinking of my weak points, I dwelt upon my good qualities. Just like God said, "It is good," I also started appreciating myself. The self-appreciation led to self-confidence, and I began to believe that I *can* do more.

When I heard that I had cancer, I wondered how it would be for society to view me as a weak woman who was now "sick." I would be viewed as a member of a separate group; a member of the weaker part of society. This thought brought a lot of pain, inferiority, and low self-esteem. I brought this terrible thought to God, and He strengthened me with His Word: *"Greetings, you who are highly favored! The Lord is with you" (Luke 1:28)*. Originally, this encouragement was given by God's angel to Mary, the mother of Jesus. She was with child, unmarried, and had to face all of society with the news of her pregnancy before marriage. Even though it was God-ordained, not many people would believe that story of a virgin carrying a child. God knew that, so he approached the young virgin with this statement: *"you who are highly favored."* God chose Mary to bear the Savior of the world out of wedlock with a divine conception because Mary was highly favored.

This is how I saw the reason for my cancer. It was because I was highly favored. God favored me! I did not have to be embarrassed of how society would view me because He showed me through His Word that He favored me! I am not supposed to be bogged down with the burden of my sickness; rather, I am supposed to be heavily filled with the favor of God. I began to dream dreams of living fearlessly, proclaiming the Word of God courageously, and accomplishing great feats with skills I never cultivated, like writing a book. The dreams led me to know deep within that despite my lack of training and proficiency, I would be able to shoulder more responsibilities without feeling weighed down. He replaced my grueling burdens with extensive favor. I rejoiced like the psalmist who said, *"How abundant are the good things that you have stored up for those who fear you, that you bestow in the sight of all, on those who take refuge in you"* (Psalm 31:19). I believed that God would exalt me in the same way He exalted Joshua: *"Today I will begin to exalt you in the eyes of all Israel, so they may know that I am with you as I was with Moses"* (Joshua 3:7). I trusted that He would magnify me the way He magnified Joshua. *"That day the LORD exalted Joshua in the sight of all Israel"* (Joshua 4:14).

I saw that God's blessings were chasing me, so I decided that I would be willing to deal with the cancer. I did not focus on the short time period of the sickness and its side effects. I turned my eyes to the future and looked forward to the exciting new future that God had planned for me after my pruning. I would not always be a cancer patient. God was opening new doors for me and I felt confident.

No one will be rejected because of his/her inabilities or weaknesses. God is the friend of the weak, so the productivity of the weak becomes more excellent and more productive than the productivity of the strong and able. When this type of belief was instilled in me, my self-confidence grew; I believed that I could actually accomplish more than the average person.

Before my sickness, I used to believe people when they said that something was difficult or hard to learn. I was fearful, so I remained small and insignificant in my ignorance and believed the negativity. Society tends to feed us more negative messages than positive. I decided for myself that I would no longer listen or believe the negativity. Instead, I would believe the opposite and choose to believe that anything is possible.

Numbers 13:33 gives the final outlook that the disbelieving and fearful Israelites had about the land into which they were finally able to set foot. While Caleb had a positive outlook and believed that they could take possession of the land, the fearful did not believe; they thought they would be overpowered. They believed they were like grasshoppers compared to the giants in the land. Because they thought of themselves as small grasshoppers, they actually wanted to turn back and leave the land that God had finally delivered to them after wandering around for forty years!

Whenever we see our difficulties in view of our own strength, rather than committing to the great arm of God, we *will* feel like grasshoppers.

While I was sick, I had people visit me with tears running down their faces and offering me sympathetic responses dripping with fear. Their words to me were not comforting or encouraging. The words were gloomy and filled with dread. I began to understand that they were extremely fearful of death and cancer, and they saw me as a sheep going out to the slaughter.

In the back of my head, I kept hearing that I would be doing great things. I knew that God had a great plan for me and that I had much to accomplish, so I had no desire to hear the sympathies of the fearful. Toward the end of my sickness, I had to stop visitors from coming because I no longer could sit and listen to their anxieties. I needed to be like the tiny frog that made it.

The Story about the Tiny Frogs

There once was a bunch of tiny frogs that arranged a race. The goal was to reach the top of a very high tower. A big crowd had gathered around the tower to see the race and cheer on the contestants.

The race began. No one in the crowd really believed that the tiny frogs would reach the top of the tower. People made statements like: "Oh, WAY too difficult!" "They will NEVER make it to the top." The tiny frogs began collapsing. The crowd continued to yell, "It is too difficult! No one will make it!" **More tiny frogs got tired and gave up** . . . But ONE continued higher and higher and higher. This one wouldn't give up! He was the only one that reached the top! All of the other tiny frogs naturally wanted to know how this one frog managed to do it. A contestant asked the tiny frog how he had found the strength to succeed and reach the goal.

It turned out that the winner was DEAF! The wisdom of this story:

- Never listen to other people's tendencies to be negative or pessimistic. They take your most

wonderful dreams and wishes away from you—
the ones you have in your heart!
- Always think of the power words have.
  Everything you hear and read will affect your
  actions!
- BE POSITIVE! And above all, be DEAF when
  people tell you that you cannot fulfill your
  dreams. Always think, *I can do this!*

No matter where you are—work, church, school, the train station—I found that we are influenced highly by negative people. I decided that I did not want those kinds of thoughts to influence me. God gave me faith in the Word of God. From Him, I have received much healing. Whoever desires, can receive from Him without reservation.

The Bible shows that those who God called to be leaders all had their own weaknesses. No one had great credentials. Moses had stuttering problems; David was the youngest and was even overlooked by his own father; Peter denied Christ; and Paul was a zealot against Christians.

"But God chose the foolish things of the world to shame the wise; God chose the weak things of the world to shame the strong" (1 Corinthians 1:27).

Acts 1:8 says, "But you will receive power when the Holy Spirit comes on you; and you will be my witnesses in Jerusalem, and in all Judea and Samaria, and to the ends of the earth." Although Peter was a simple fisherman by trade, when the Holy Spirit descended on him, he was able to speak so powerfully that he brought almost three thousand people to salvation. The Holy Spirit is a promise that is given to those who long eagerly for it. God does not look at our past. When we go to God and repent of our sins, He forgives us and fills us with the power of the Holy Spirit.

If you think small, you will be small. If you think big, you will be big. So focus on the positive and stay determined. As Joel Osteen says, God believes in you even more than you believe in yourself.

Discovering My Inner Talents

The culture of India in the 1970s highly regarded the teaching profession. A teacher was highly esteemed, and I had great desires to become a teacher and receive the accolades that came with a teaching degree.

As an aspiring teacher, I attended college and received my Bachelors of Education, with honors, in 1974. The ranking was based on how well a student performed in theory and in practical application. For the practical part, students were required to teach a high-school class for a month and be observed by college professors and the principal. Even though I was pregnant with my first child, I performed well and was considered to be the highest ranked teacher in my class of one hundred students, which meant that I taught at the student's level, was knowledgeable in the subject matter, was able to teach complex subjects in simple ways, carried myself with confidence, and respected my students. However in order to be awarded with this honor, I would have to observed by the commissioner as well and get his approval.

The presentation before the commissioner was scheduled for March 15, but my due date was March 13. Being empathetic to my condition, my principal asked me to provide all of my records and credentials so that he could recommend me by word to the commissioner. On that day in early March, my membrane ruptured, and I started leaking fluid. I ended up in the hospital for ten days before finally going through labor and delivering my first child, who was extremely malnourished. Because of the leak, she ended up dying within a few days of her birth. Not only was I unable to present before the commissioner to receive my high ranking, but I now had a great sorrow that had developed within me. Thankfully, my husband was thoughtful enough to gather all my papers and deliver them to the principal. Unfortunately, because I could not physically be present for evaluation, I was given second class. I still had to deal with the loss of my child and face the embarrassment and pressure of going back to my husband's home with no child in tow.

Thankfully, the family encouraged me rather than frowning upon me. Within three months of all of this happening, I received a call from my principal asking me to give a "model class" to the B. Ed (Bachelor of Education) students for that year. I remember how delightful that news was in light of my recent sorrows and disappointments. My husband pushed me to participate and even joked with me saying that he would be sitting in that room as well. With this opportunity, I was able to use my God-given talent—unknown to me at that time—to help others.

Due to my husband's work relocation, we had to move to Dubai in the United Arab Emirites where I worked as a housewife caring for our two children. My aspirations were set aside due to the needs of my children and my talents were hidden deep within.

In 1982, we moved to the United States. Because we could not live off my husband's meager income, I was forced to work, but America was different from India. I did not speak the English language fluently, I did not know the culture, and I was afraid to pursue my teaching career. I wanted a job where I did not have to stand in front of people, so I went back to college to get a degree to practice medical technology. That time of my life was very difficult. We were in a foreign country and had limited resources trying to make life work. I had to work, care for my children, and go to college all at the same time. By the grace of God, I survived and graduated. Rather than pursue a career, I simply looked for a job that would pay the bills. I worked just as an employee and not as a goal-oriented person with a vision behind her. I looked for the least stressful position. I worked as a medical technologist, raised my children, and cared for my husband. I was mediocre. Although I came to America with the knowledge of my exemplary teaching skill, I did not pursue it because of my own fears, which limited me. I did not want to contribute anything to the company because I convinced myself that the life I was struggling through would be enough. I did not want to dream. I was an enemy to myself.

In the year 2000, my supervisor gave his group the chance to become certified in a particular area of microbiology. I did not have the self-motivation to do this. A co-worker, who was also a foreigner, encouraged me to go because she did not want to attend by herself. Wanting to keep her company, I participated. We both took the class and received our certification. Although my co-worker had a desire to do the job, I was very hesitant. For seventeen years, I had worked in the same position hearing the others explain how difficult the job was and how it required a certain skill level and education level. It was ingrained in me that only the high-performing employees could complete that task well. Certainly, I was not qualified. I chose to believe all the negative thoughts.

Soon after, a new director, Jim Adams, came into the picture. He was a man who believed in hard work, was very determined, thought positive, and gave opportunities for his employees to grow. His thoughts would often be quoted in our local newsletters. Reading his articles influenced my thoughts and made me realize that I should not stay where I was; I should grow. Jim Adams brought great change to our environment.

One change he wanted to make was to transfer all of our paper-based test procedures online. The procedures were currently contained in folders that were kept around the lab, but they were not kept up to date and needed to be rewritten. He simply instructed all of the lab workers that rewriting the procedure was a task that needed to be completed, and he gave us a deadline. This was the push that I needed. I remembered an article he wrote in our interdepartmental newsletter: he challenged us to become more than employees who came in merely to get a paycheck. I thought that although I had faithfully served my company for seventeen years, no one would ever remember me when I left. On the other hand, with this opportunity to rewrite a procedure, my name could remain as the author of a practice for some time to come. In this way, I could give back to my lab community. So I authored the procedure, and it brought great confidence in my abilities and pride in my work—something that was lacking before.

Another change that was going to be implemented was transferring some of my work over to the lab support group, who would need to be trained. I was reminded of my ability to teach, so I volunteered. Teaching the class would require me to use a PowerPoint presentation. I had never used PowerPoint, but I looked at it as an opportunity to learn something new. With help from my daughters and co-workers, I was able to create an excellent presentation, for which I was given a great review.

I had been working seventeen years in this position, but I had never dared to step foot outside of my comfort zone, and no one knew about my hidden talents. I realized sadly that I had not pushed myself to excel. After my cancer, however, all of the cowardice, lack of desire, and laziness transformed into eagerness to outperform, boldness, and a desire to work hard. The reason I wanted to excel after my experience with cancer was because I was determined to not allow anyone to view me as a weak part of society.

When it came to giving the in-service to the lab group, I had some hesitation. My negative thoughts came back and plagued me: Would I be able to present clearly with my broken English? Would I know enough to teach well? I went home and brought my weaknesses before God during my quiet time. I laid down all of my hesitations before His feet, and He encouraged me with a Word: *"Then how is it that each of us hears them in our own native language?" (Acts 2:8).*

This verse is part of a passage in Acts where the Holy Spirit came down on the day of Pentecost; although there were people of multiple nations and tongues present, each man could understand the other—nothing short of a miracle of God. In the same way, God encouraged me with Acts 2:8, allowing me to take faith in the fact that God would enable my broken English to be understood by all the people who were attending the class.

So with faith, I presented yet another class. Not only did

everyone understand my accent and teaching, but they complimented my class and I was asked to give yet another one!

This process brought incredible joy to my soul and gave me motivation to work hard yet again. I wanted to move forward. I felt that God was searching me out. When God's favor is upon us, we receive it all! Those who ask for an unselfish need and have a desire to help others will receive all the gifts necessary to accomplish that need; it is given through faith. When God's favor rests on us, we become capable and inferiority leaves. God's strength and God's wisdom is much greater than man's, so through Him we are able to achieve far greater than what we could on our own. There is no limitation with sickness or with disability; when we finally decide to take a step of faith, when we decide to go the extra mile, God's divine providence rests on our paths.

After my sickness, I evaluated myself and noticed that I always took the path of least resistance. I never wanted to hone my skills or take any risks. I only wanted what came easy. A bishop who lived in the nineteenth century, Philips Brooks, said not to pray for a comfortable life but pray instead to receive strength to handle all that life throws our way. Jesus said the same thing: *"Whoever wants to be my disciple must deny themselves and take up their cross daily and follow me" (Luke 9:23)*. The Bible does not promise a comfortable life, but it does promise that God will strengthen you, and it encourages you not to fear. It says that those who are weak will be strengthened by His Holy Spirit. That is the great promise of the Holy Spirit, and it is faith in His strength combined with our willingness to work hard that brings us to success.

This value can be found in the story of the eagle that refused to fly:[6]

---

[6] Story found on http://www.manoramaonline.com/cgi-bin/ MMOnline.dll/portal/ep/malayalamContentView.do?contentId=1 2057955&programId=1073753694&BV_ID=@@@&channelId=-1073751705&tabId=9 ,posted 25 July 2012.

Because of its powerful body and ability to fly higher than other birds, the eagle has earned its reputation as the king of birds. These birds are a common sight in the Arabian Gulf countries. People use these birds for entertainment and competition. Once, the ruler of an Arabian country received two eagles as a gift; they were a dominant species. They had beautiful bodies and beaks that were sharper than a sword and were interesting to interact with. The king entrusted a bird trainer to help train the birds.

After several months, the king asked for the eagles. The trainer came back and said to the king, "One of the birds is an excellent roamer; he is as fast as a jet plane. Unfortunately, the other one refuses to move from the tree branch, which he is settled in. From the day that he found the branch, he avoids risking the task of flying." The king was sorely disappointed. He brought in researchers and trainers around the country but all failed in getting the bird to move. He even appointed a magician to no avail. Finally, the king thought it might be smart to get a local farmer involved. Soon, he ordered the palace keeper to bring a farmer to the castle. Without much delay, the farmer was brought to the palace and informed about the king's dilemma. The following day, the king got a surprising message that the eagle, which once refused to move from his comfortable tree branch, was now soaring high in the sky. He himself witnessed the eagle's flight. On questioning the farmer about the secret of this eagle's transformation, the farmer with utmost humility told the king, "Oh dear king, that was a very simple thing that I did; I cut off the branch on which the eagle perched and now it is forced to fly."

We are all destined to soar high like this eagle; the Almighty has given ample talents and abilities to accomplish such a goal. Unfortunately, many people are comfortable on their tried and true perches; they do not want to fly from that branch because it is enough. So, sometimes God will break off that branch so that we learn to soar. In my case, I had a desire twenty-one years ago to help cancer patients, but it did not come to fruition. To fulfill that desire, God allowed me to go through cancer and pushed me to a place where I could truly offer help to others. It no longer stopped at desire; rather, the desire has now come to life. Although the push from God was initially painful, I see now that the push was well worth the outcome.

When I was young, I lived in comfort without any sickness or difficulties presented to me. I lived in comfort without any sickness or difficulties presented to me. So when I received the news of my cancer, it brought incredible shock and distress to my soul. I was in such agony that I had to call out to God; I realized that no human being could really help me. The Psalmist said, *"It is better to take refuge in the Lord than to trust in humans" (Psalm 118:8).* I let go of everything that I had ever put my hope in, everything that I desired, and when I became empty, I yearned for God's presence. Daily, I sought out His divine presence. I wanted God so badly to impress Himself upon me. I wanted to live solely by His Holy Spirit. When I sought Him out, He came to me. When He came to me, my faith became stronger, and I lost the fear of my cancer. I knew that His most powerful presence was within me, even more powerful than cancer. When I realized WHO it was that was living inside of me, I lost all fear of sickness, I lost fear of death, and I lost any anxieties residing in me. I literally had the power of the living God in me. I was unstoppable. My faith became so strong that I believed, no, *knew*, that I could claim victory over anything that came my way.

I volunteer with the Cancer Society and have the chance to talk to many women who have recently found out about their cancer. I can now understand the hopelessness, anxiety, and depression some of them are facing. I asked God to do to them what He did to me— relieve them of their fears and anxieties and to bring them to a place of hope. What I experienced was that the more I prayed for others, the more strength I was given. Their burdens became my burdens. I cried for these women who were not my relatives. I burdened myself with their needs the same way that Nehemiah burdened himself with his people's needs.

Nehemiah was a man of God who worked in the king's palace as a wine server to the king. Though he lived in the king's courts and suffered no hardships, Nehemiah knew that his own people were suffering, and he himself became very troubled. The king noticed Nehemiah's disposition and asked him to give the reason for his depression. Nehemiah took the opportunity to request the king's favor in helping the Jews rebuild the wall of Jerusalem. Once he received permission and started building, he was ridiculed by many, but he tolerated the vast persecution because he knew that rebuilding the city walls were important. Nehemiah was a man who bore the mockery of the people because of his passion toward them.

Nehemiah's experience touched me and gave me the motivation to write this book. In the same way that he took the burden of his people, I saw the needs of cancer patients around me, and I could sense their pain. Sometimes, the pain was intolerable and their pain became my pain. I wanted to share my experience with others. I wanted them to see how God would deliver them from the snare in which they had been caught. He would give them a strength that was unshakable, a hope that could not be extinguished, talents that would be honed, courage to withstand criticism, and a spirit that offered forgiveness and grace. The spirit of grace is the most precious gift that I have ever received in my entire life. Living with grace and offering forgiveness brings the person to a position of great power. I wish I had this type of spirit when I was young.

Fight to Advance

Many people, when faced with failures, life-threatening sicknesses, or family death, experience depression and sometimes even desire to quit. Fear grips their ability to fight and move forward. While going through chemo, my oncologist told me that the perseverance and faith of a person was often tested during this time. Inside, I knew that I had been delivered from a grand mal seizure at one time in my life, and I would be delivered from this disease as well. Even though I had some fears about the seizure that occurred ten years prior to my cancer, I had been relieved from those fears. Enduring adversity and hardship develops strength because it is during our points of utter weakness that we realize our shortcomings and are forced to rely on the strength of God. When this divine strength is experienced, we crave it more and more.

King Philip enrolled his child into a Greek public school. At a very young age, his son, Alexander, was forced into manual labor and was faced with hardships and oppression. The school required three years of this grueling curriculum. Some kids would run away because they could not handle the rigor. But King Philip's goal was for his son to overcome these difficulties. After the first three years, the students were required to take a test in fire. The children were given cast iron bowls filled with hot coals and were asked to hold it in the palm of their hands. The test was to hold the hot bowls in their palms for a few hours without wincing. During Alexander's day of testing, the king and queen—his father and mother—came to witness the test. While Alexander was holding the bowl, a piece of coal burst from the heat and fell onto his bare leg, burning the flesh. When his mother, the queen, saw the incident, she rushed forward to rescue her baby. But the king, Alexander's father, held her back saying, "What do you know? I am raising him as a strong man." The boy raised with this type of rigor turned out to be Alexander the Great.

Success in life and in spirituality comes only by withstanding discomforts, misfortunes, and tragedies. James 1:12 says, *"Blessed is the one who perseveres under trial because, having stood the test, that person will receive the crown of life that the Lord has promised to those who love him."* Experiencing trials is a privilege because we are not alone. He who is able to strengthen you lives within you. I experienced this. After losing my hair and nails, enduring nausea, sitting through long periods of chemo, being unable to eat properly, and losing an entire breast, I felt that I had passed the test of fire. When I finally reentered the world, I presented myself with joy and not with sorrow. I entered the world as a new woman filled with strength and not as a weak cancer patient.

Suffering can elicit one of two different emotions in people. Some will draw away from God, filled with bitterness and anger. Others will draw near to Him, with trust and confidence. I chose to draw near to God, so I received more confidence. I received an ability I never had before—to face responsibility. I used to run from responsibility, fearing failure. But after my experience with God, I realized that spirituality was not just about worship; it was about receiving strength to do the impossible and to conquer fears.

Rather than complaining about my situation, I fought it with a positive attitude and trust in God. I realized that life was just getting shorter and that I had less time to accomplish what was in store for me in the future. I felt regret that I had not done more for God or for my community so far in life. Although I had many talents, I hid them due to fear, laziness, and a desire for comfort. Although I claimed to have faith, I never acted out my faith.

The good news was that God changed me. He transformed me. I only heard about God in the past, but during my cancer, I actually experienced God. Today, there is an inner strength that bursts forth from within, a spirit that liberates me to perform with a greater measure of vigor than I have ever known before.

Because I held so much regret about my past, I became very sensitive to this issue in other people's lives. A great surge of holy anger dwells within when I see young men and women wasting their talents because of fear or because of ignorance. When I see people avoiding responsibility, not wanting to stray from their comfort zone, I start praying for them. My hope is that if they receive strong faith at a young age, they will be able to do many seemingly difficult and impossible things for God.

Now, as a cancer survivor, I have determined in my heart not to allow my sickness or age to be a limitation to my outlook on life. Of course, I do live with a life-threatening disease. This is a fact. But I choose to live acknowledging the favor of God in my life. I believe and have faith that Christ's power rests on me in my time of weakness. I feel like Caleb in the Bible when he said, *"I am still as strong today as the day Moses sent me out; I'm just as vigorous to go out to battle now as I was then. Now give me this hill country that the LORD promised me that day. You yourself heard then that the Anakites were there and their cities were large and fortified, but, the LORD helping me, I will drive them out just as he said"* (Joshua 14:11–12). Caleb was eighty-five years old when he made this statement. Age was no barrier for this courageous man of strong faith. Rather than focusing on his weaknesses and old age, he focused on the strength of God. In the same way, I also started to look at God as my strength rather than relying on my own abilities or on my own flesh. I also started to encourage my husband, who was close to retirement age. We desire now for God to keep us busy during our old age. We do not desire to sit at home in safety and lack of excitement.

This is our prayer: *"Now to him who is able to do immeasurably more than all we ask or imagine, according to his power that is at work within us"* (Ephesians 3:20).

When our understanding of God increases, faith grows and self-confidence is increased. Through our struggles, we mature; battles invigorate strength and cultivate skill.

Teach us to number our days.
(Psalm 90:12)

*M*oses, the deliverer of the Jews, cried out in Psalm 90:12: *"Teach us to number our days, that we may gain a heart of wisdom."* In our youth, we think we will live forever, so we do not understand the value of time. Life is like a book; with every turn of the page, you get closer to death. We do not have much time, and we allow time to pass without doing all the things that matter.

Who am I? How many years or days will I live? There is also a day and time for us to face the judgment seat of God, but we do not consider those things. It is as Solomon said, *"and the dust returns to the ground it came from, and the spirit returns to God who gave it" (Ecclesiastes 12:7).*

Saint Alphonsa, who started out as a sister in the convent, went through many trials in her life. In one of her books, she stated that a day without a trial makes her feel empty. When we expect comfort and ease in life, we set ourselves up for regret and failure, and that's what brings us depression. It is important to change that type of thinking and to understand what the reality of life offers. We are all dying, whether or not you are a cancer patient. With every breath of life, we are one step closer to death. When no diagnosis of sickness is given, no value is given to each day of life. When the diagnosis is given, the reality of life's impermanence settles in, and you begin to realize that life is precious and time is precious.

Life on earth is not permanent for anyone. Doctor. Patient. Healthy people. Sick folks. The rich. The poor. All will die. There is no way to live forever on earth. Seventy or eighty years is the average life span. That is a very short period of time to live. Those who lived before us have already left. After some time, we also will leave. When we understand this fact, we will manage our time, talents, and treasure, especially time. Spend your time wisely.

Death is a reality, but most of us do not want to think of death. While we are living, we are dying actually. All see death with fear. But Revelation 14:13 says, *"Then I heard a voice from heaven say, 'Write this: Blessed are the dead who die in the Lord from now on.' 'Yes,' says the Spirit, 'they will rest from their labor, for their deeds will follow them.'"*

Every day is a gift from God. On our own, we have nothing. We are simply the keepers of all that have been given to us. No one has brought anything into this world and no one can take anything out of this world. It is when we count our days that we are able to become good stewards of all that is given to us. When we count our days, we will receive a heart of gratitude. Selfishness will be removed, and we will learn to share ourselves, our money, and our talent with others. Tomorrow does not belong to us. We may want to put things off for tomorrow, but we do not know what tomorrow will hold. As it says in scripture, *"I tell you, now is the time of God's favor, now is the day of salvation"* (2 Corinthians 6:2).

Jesus said in John 9:4, *"As long as it is day, we must do the works of him who sent me. Night is coming, when no one can work."* I understand this to mean that our capacity in life will slowly diminish. We will not be able to do as much as we could in our younger days. If, in our young age, we could have counted our days, we would have made great investments here on earth and in heaven. Everything that we own is temporary. If a man gains the world but does not gain his soul, what is the point? Somehow, we constantly ignore our soul and our soul cries out from within. John 3:3 says we must be born again. It is when we are born again that we will receive eternity in heaven.

We should invest in eternity. When we do, we can receive joy knowing that what lies there is much better than what we live in or live with today. Our life on earth is filled with sickness and tears, but life in heaven is free of tears and sickness. We should work for that eternity, for our salvation.

For our light and momentary troubles are achieving for us an eternal glory that far outweighs them all. So we fix our eyes not on what is seen, but on what is unseen, since what is seen is temporary, but what is unseen is eternal (2 Corinthians 4:17–18).

So, how do we invest in our eternity? The book of Matthew gives us clear instruction.

"For I was hungry and you gave me something to eat, I was thirsty and you gave me something to drink, I was a stranger and you invited me in, I needed clothes and you clothed me, I was sick and you looked after me, I was in prison and you came to visit me" (Matthew 25:35–36).

Matthew 25 tells us the parable of the talents (money). A man going on a journey called his servants and gave his goods to him. To one, he gave five talents, to another two talents, and to a third, the man gave him one talent. The servant who was given five talents increased his share by another five. The servant who was given two talents increased it by another two. But the servant who was given one talent dug it into the ground and did not even try to make an increase. So when the man returned, he was pleased with his first two servants but greatly displeased with the third. He took the talent from the servant who was given one and gave it to the servant who had ten.

Just like Moses said, when we get the wisdom to count our days then we will:

- procrastinate no longer
- increase our talents
- develop a fear and reverence of God

From this fear of God, we will gain the desire to do good for others.

Most of my family was in India when I was diagnosed with cancer. When my husband notified them, I received a call from one of my cousins, Mathew. He showered me with his sympathies. He and all of my other family members saw me as a woman whose days were coming to a quick end. They saw me as a victim. Some of them cried during their phone conversations with me, and this would bring me down.

In 2008, one year after the onset of my cancer, I received word that my cousin, Mathew, had died from a massive heart attack. When Mathew heard of my cancer, he probably thought that I would die soon; I am sure he never thought once that he would be the one to pass away before me. Since my cancer diagnosis, many people around me have died. Some were younger than me, some older. Some had cancer; some had none. Some died in a car accident and others died of old age. This helped me to see that cancer and death really had no direct correlation.

Death is a reality. However, our lives will not end until our heavenly Father calls us home. My cousin Mathew's time was up because God had determined it so. My time continues. When cancer is first announced to a new patient, he will go through many different emotions: anger, depression, fear, etc. Fear was my biggest enemy. I remember that I had purchased a book to learn about breast cancer, and the last chapter talked about death. I was so scared that I never allowed myself to even turn to that page. I soon realized that I had great fear of death. I realized that I was not prepared for death or judgment. Realizing this doubt can bring great fear. Many people face this type of fear because the news is given suddenly, without any warning. No one thinks of where he was and where he might be going.

All of us were born with a two-way ticket; we come from God and we are to go back to God. But most of the time, unfortunately, we do not think that way. Because of life's business or because of our lack of hope of eternity, we do not think of this great need to go back to God. Life is lived only once. We cannot turn back to the path already traveled. We will not always be in this present life either. So the life that you live should be lived with the utmost care. We should use our abilities and skills to share with others and to enrich our community. God gave us certain talents and put us on this earth for just a short time. It is up to us how we decide to live that life. God has also given us a time period for how long we will live on this earth. When the time is up, God will call us. Since we do not know when that time is, we should always be prepared to meet our Maker.

We are the keepers of our time, and when God calls us

and asks us to give an account of our lives, we should be able to give a reasonable account. Our lives are not meant to be lived with carelessness. This world is not our final home. Our journey should be toward an eternity in heaven.

In facing fear, I used to meditate on First and Second Corinthians. These books described the amazing courage of Paul. Though he fought Christ in his past, he had since been given an incredible change of character and faced death with fearlessness. I asked God to give me that type of outlook on death. I did not want to fear it; I wanted to conquer it.

According to Buddhist wisdom, one learns to truly live only when death knocks at the door. When I learned of my cancer, it was sudden shock into reality. I realized that I only had a few years left to live. The Bible says that a man only has seventy or eighty years of good living, after which comes suffering and finally death. At the time of my diagnosis, I was already in my mid-fifties. Only by removing the fear of death could I live the rest of my life victoriously. I decided that I also wanted a peaceful death. I did not want to die with fear and trepidation: I wanted to die acknowledging my time and accepting my eternity.

In 2 Kings 20:1, it is said of King Hezekiah: *"In those days Hezekiah became ill and was at the point of death. The prophet Isaiah son of Amoz went to him and said, 'This is what the LORD says: Put your house in order, because you are going to die; you will not recover.'"* Death comes to all; it does not discriminate. Moses prayed this prayer in Psalm 90:12: *"Teach us to number our days, that we may gain a heart of wisdom."*

But the great thing is that though my body may pass away, the deeds I have done for others will live on. Though my flesh will pass, the fruitful thoughts I have released to those around me will linger. I resolved not to live any longer with the fear of death. Living with cancer means that you have to face death every day, but I did not want to face death with dread. I determined in my heart to change this thought pattern and to live out my life, facing death, from a standpoint of victory.

The Bible gives many promises of life after death. When I feared death, it was because I did not fully comprehend or believe the promises of eternity in heaven. In 1986, when my father was close to death, my entire family was in denial. No one would talk about it, but we all knew he was close to death. I was scared of talking about the subject, much less pray about it. How I wish that I had the knowledge twenty years ago that I have today.

After death, we live with God for an eternity. *"And the dust returns to the ground it came from, and the spirit returns to God who gave it" (Ecclesiastes 12:7)*. To attain this, we should live with God so that we can die with God. In my fifty-sixth year of life, I finally started to live with God, and He gave me an incredible transformation so that I became fearless. Rather than dreading death and focusing on when the end of my life would come, I started to live with passion, doing things with purpose. I stopped complaining and started rejoicing. Today it seems that I enjoy life so much more than I did prior to cancer.

Yearning for a holy heart and a steadfast spirit, I cry out to God to keep me from turning to the lusts of my flesh. With daily meditation, I am able to maintain a heart of forgiveness and a spirit that is faithful. The cry of my heart is to live victoriously here on earth *and* in heaven. That is God's desire, as well.

When I go to work, I take the train. When I come back home, I take the train. The ride back home is filled with people relieved that their workday has ended, and they can go back home, to the place they love, the place that is waiting to receive them with joy. In the same way, we are created and sent to the world, and then we die and are sent back to the place from where we were created. When we return home to the Creator, we should go with joy in our hearts, knowing that He is waiting to receive us with joy.

One day on the train, this lady, who I had seen on a regular basis, seemed giddy and happy, different from most days. When I inquired of her glee, she said that her boss was not going to be in that day. Because he would not be there, she could do what she wanted. Quite often, this is how we live our lives. We do things carelessly thinking no one is watching. But the truth is that there is One who knows our very thoughts, not just the things we actually do. When we discern God's watchful eye, we should become stewards of our time and talents. Think about how much you could have accomplished up to this point in your life had you been aware of God's accountability.

Many people live with no goals. In my work place, we are given evaluations every year. If all we have done in that entire year is the minimum job requirement, our maximum pay increase is 2 percent. But if we have gone above and beyond and can prove it, then we are qualified to receive a higher raise or promotion. At work, we are also required to write down our goals for the next year. Then we work toward accomplishing those goals and show at the end of the year how well we performed.

In life, I have also learned to set goals and work hard at accomplishing those goals. My life before cancer was lived with a carefree attitude, not worrying about what I could supply to the world around me. But after cancer, I began to notice everything with a thoughtful eye. From the computers I worked on to the towels I dried myself with—all were created for the benefit of society. But what had I done to contribute? Nothing. After cancer, I decided to set goals for myself and do things with purpose. I did not want this realization of all of the time and talents that I have wasted to be for nothing; I wanted others who were younger than me to learn from my mistakes. Writing this book is part of my contribution to society. My hope is that others can learn from my mistakes and alter their future by it.

I have also learned to give thanks every day for the little things in life. I have learned to enjoy the small joys of life. I have learned to desire to be excellent at work and to give my 110 percent to life. I realized that the fear of death will do nothing but stop success. So I learned to accept the fact that death is just another part of life. My focus would not be on death; rather, it would be on life and living it to the fullest.

At a young age, while living in India in the mid-sixties I was asked by my father one rainy morning to make coffee for him. Not wanting to deny him, I obediently, but reluctantly, went to the stove. Now, our stove in India in the sixties was nothing like the stoves we cook on in modern America. The fire had to be lighted manually. The stove was comprised of a brick layer topped with wood. Once a fire had been ignited and used for cooking, ashes were left behind. It was on this type of stove on which I tried to make coffee. Without cleaning the ashes, I tried and tried to strike a fire but to no avail. It was impossible to create a fire unless the ashes were first cleaned. But I was lazy, not wanting to dirty my hands, so I tried over and over in vain to create this fire. Our relationship to God and our existence with sin and regret is similar to lighting a fire over an unclean stove. Our regrets and sins are the ashes on the hearth; it is important to clean out the ashes and remove them from the stove before we can light the fire of the Holy Spirit.

I created a habit that helped me to clean out the ashes. Although my husband and I pray every morning together, I began to meditate by myself for about fifteen minutes every day prior to our prayer time. I would take verses from the Bible and focus just on what the message was, removing all other thoughts from my head. As I continued to do this on a daily basis, I saw a transformation in myself; I began to be filled with joy. I was turning into a new creation; the old was passing away. Meditation was incredibly powerful, and it brought incredible joy. It also filled me with extreme faith.

One day as I was talking to a very successful businesswoman, I noticed that she seemed very sad. She told me with tears in her eyes of the guilt she was carrying around. She was an older woman with grown children, and she was not sure if she had been a good mother or not. I explained to her that God can renew all things and that if she could come to a place of acknowledgment, God would forgive her and give her a new heart. After David repented of his horrible sin of adultery and murder, he received forgiveness from God. Then, out of a sense of relief, he proclaimed in Psalm 32:1, *"Blessed is the one whose transgressions are forgiven, whose sins are covered."* God forgives all of our transgressions, but we have to believe, repent, and receive the forgiveness. We have to humble ourselves, throw away our pride, and acknowledge ourselves as sinners. Then we have to return to God and ask Him to forgive us. We have to acknowledge our need for Him, come humbly before His presence, and ask Him to forgive us. When we come to this point in our lives, God looks at us with a Father's compassion, and He yearns to help us out of our dilemma. We will receive incredible healing and unbelievable joy.

To be healed from physical infirmities, we rely on a physician. To receive spiritual healing, we rely on God. Both are important. Both are necessary. If you are sick, do not just seek physical healing; seek spiritual healing as well. You will feel much more complete and receive much more joy.

When I came into this type of faith, all of my thoughts changed. All of my mind's stresses were relieved. I received the capacity to forgive others freely. What an awesome gift. *Jesus replied, "Very truly I tell you, no one can see the kingdom of God unless they are born again" (John 3:3).* I am a new creation. Even those around me comment on my transformation. They say that my face shines now.

My husband and I attended a church conference recently. There were eight hundred people there. As the bishop preached, I began to think that he had no idea who I was. He had no idea of my difficulties or what I had been through. God, however, knew me. He knows exactly how many hairs are on my head, and He knows the exact thoughts that I think daily. He knows me, and I know Him. But the world's leaders and spiritual leaders are only human; they cannot possibly know everyone they serve.

Luke 10:20 says, *"However, do not rejoice that the spirits submit to you, but rejoice that your names are written in heaven."* This verse gave me amazing joy. My fears of death were vanquished because I realized that my name was written in heaven. I want to live the rest of my life with extreme faith. Rather than allowing the difficulties of life to bring me down, I know that I have a God who is with me every step of the way.

During his lifetime, King David had to face the deaths of many people who were close to him, three of whom I would like to focus on. Two were the deaths of his own children and one was the death of the commander in chief of King Saul, a rival to David.

The first child's death was a result of God punishing David for the adultery he committed with Bathsheba and the murder he carried out on her husband. When a prophet confronted David of his sin, David knelt before God and fasted for several days, hoping for mercy to see his child live. But when he saw that God did not oblige and that the child passed away, he stopped his fast, put on lively clothes, and began to live life again. Everyone around him was confused and when they asked why he fasted while the child was sick but rejoiced now that he had passed away, David replied, *"While the child was still alive, I fasted and wept. I thought, 'Who knows? The LORD may be gracious to me and let the child live.' But now that he is dead, why should I go on fasting? Can I bring him back again? I will go to him, but he will not return to me"* (2 Samuel 12:22–23). David held fast to hope.

The second death was of his child, Absalom, who was much older and who had declared war against his father, David, trying to gain his throne. Even though David agreed to the battle, he had a soft spot in his heart for his child and asked his soldiers to have mercy if they ever had to face Absalom in battle. But in the midst of the battle, Absalom was put to death. When David heard of his son's passing, he went into a state of depression and mourned out loud for his son. Even though his own son was his enemy, his heart was greatly troubled by the son's death. There was no hope in this death. It was a hopeless cry.

The third death was of Abner, the commander in chief of Saul's army, who had left King Saul and went to serve King David. A great bond and relationship had formed between Abner and David. So when Abner was treacherously killed in battle, David showed a sincere and profound sorrow; he publicly mourned and fasted to honor the death of this great man. Abner's was a wretched death.

The deaths of Absalom and Abner grieved King David. The memory of their lives brought pain. Absalom's death, in particular, brought pain because the memory of the son was of the uprising he sought. There was no peace in the thoughts of Absalom, only opposition and destruction. Eternity was questionable in their deaths. But when Bathsheba's son died, there was great hope that David would yet again see his son in heaven. This hope is what brought celebration into the time of the son's death.

When we live with Jesus and die with Jesus, our lives become a testimony for others. Our testimony becomes hope for others. Just like David believed that he would see his son yet again, they will say of the dead man that they will see him yet again in heaven.

Scripture says it well. *"Brothers and sisters, we do not want you to be uninformed about those who sleep in death, so that you do not grieve like the rest of mankind, who have no hope. For we believe that Jesus died and rose again, and so we believe that God will bring with Jesus those who have fallen asleep in him. According to the Lord's word, we tell you that we who are still alive, who are left until the coming of the Lord, will certainly not precede those who have fallen asleep. For the Lord himself will come down from heaven, with a loud command, with the voice of the archangel and with the trumpet call of God, and the dead in Christ will rise first. After that, we who are still alive and are left will be caught up together with them in the clouds to meet the Lord in the air. And so we will be with the Lord forever. Therefore encourage one another with these words" (1 Thessalonians 4:13–18).*

Wisdom is gained by counting the days of our lives. It helps us to exercise our time, talent, and treasure. Procrastination will change to motivation when we count our days. It helps us to remain humble in the midst of our successes. We will be filled with love, we will want to accomplish much, and we will desire to be a role model to others when we learn to count our days.

Aley, tell me why you are different from my other patients.

When I first came into the care of my oncologist, she sensed my intense fear. She knew that it was overwhelming for me and even gave me phone numbers of cancer survivors so that I could be comforted by their stories. After my chemo treatments were over, I returned to my oncologist for a routine checkup, this time with a renewed sense of hope. Dr. Lee, after observing my change of character, said to me, "Aley, tell me why you are different from my other patients." She could see that I was stress free, my face shone, and that my attitude was bright and cheery. I replied, "I am not dealing with this sickness on my own." If I were dealing with it on my own, it would be overwhelming, but because I was depending on strength from God, it became possible. I came to accept my weaknesses and relied on the power of God. I also let go of all that I used to trust in—my education, my husband, my family. I understood that help from them was limited because they were human and limited themselves. My only source of strength was God, whose power is limitless.

I also was able to rid myself of any guilt harbored from my past. I let go of the guilt that came from living with pride, from loving others more than God, and from worshipping other things before God. I let go of the guilt that came from turning my eyes away from those in need. I accepted God's forgiveness and believed that He had now transformed me to become a person who was redeemed from those things of which I was once guilty. Today, the joy that comes from meditating on His Word, living out His commands, and telling others about His goodness and love has become quite intense. Even the very thought of the love He has shown to me brings me incredible delight.

I volunteer with the American Cancer Society. When new patients arrive, I can easily understand their shock and the series of emotions they go through. I remember a time when I could not deal with the pain that came from the news of my cancer, so I now understand what these patients are going through. I often go home and pray for them, asking God to give them the same relief from fear that He gave me and to provide them with the same hope that He gave me. The interesting thing is that after I pray earnestly for my sisters, I am left feeling incredibly strengthened.

One day during my volunteer work, the surgeon who attended to me came and notified me of a newly diagnosed patient in her forties who was being very difficult. When I pulled her aside, she confided in me. Her husband was already a cancer patient. He was receiving chemotherapy and was very depressed. She was the one who was encouraging her husband. She was the one driving him to his treatments, and now she was being diagnosed with the same thing. My heart was in so much pain, but I refused to cry in front of her. At first, I was speechless. Inside, I prayed and asked God to give me a word with which I could encourage her. After I listened to her for a while, I told her that this disease was only temporary and that God would give her more strength than she ever had before. I told her not to focus on the present and to look for the good. I explained to her how God had done that for me, and He would do the same for her.

After my experience with her, I began to realize that what I had gone through (and was going through) was nothing in comparison to her circumstances. I used to wonder how I could continue to face the remnant of cancer—something I have to live with every day. But life extends out in front of me, and I do not want to be a burden to those around me. Rather, I ask God to strengthen me to help others with their difficulties. So, I meditate. On a daily basis, I focus on four specific things:

(1) Nothing is impossible for God.
(2) I can do everything through Him who gives me strength.
(3) God chose me, even as a cancer patient. Just as He searched for the donkey on which the Son of God should ride, God chose me to be a vessel to fill.
(4) I am a victor. God's favor is upon me. Even though I am weak, I become strong through Him.

These four things give me strength on a daily basis to do my best. My job requires a lot of focus and concentration. I am required to produce reports with no errors. I have to train others. When I arrive home, I have additional duties to complete. My God enables me to do all of these things.

God has filled me with the joy of His salvation.

God will not remember any of my past sins. In the midst of my sins, I went to my Savior. As I drew near to Him, He drew near to me. Today, when I consider the love and the goodness of God, it brings me great joy. As I grew closer to God and understood that God was so much bigger than all of my sin, I began to empty myself of my pride and arrogance. With that emptiness, I started to forget my past and grow toward my future.

There are many troubles in the world, but that is okay. When I was young, I desired to live a life free of troubles. I now realize that a carefree life is not a reality. In reality, are things like death, sickness, and poverty. Christ does not offer a trouble-free life; in fact, He says to take up the cross and follow Him. As I began to ponder on these thoughts, I also began to see my sickness as a minor obstacle in my life. What was in store for me was so much bigger and held so much more purpose than what I was going through. God's desire was for me to spend all of eternity with Him in heaven, free forever, with no pain, sorrow, or death. Although my troubles existed, they were no longer the focus of my life. They were just a small part of my reality.

In biblical days, Jews and Samaritans did not get along. When Jesus, who was Jewish, met the Samaritan woman by the well, He knew all of her past sins. Yet, with that knowledge, He asked her to give Him some water. The woman was so surprised that a Jewish man would speak to her, a Samaritan woman, but Jesus had no partiality toward gender, social status, or past sins. Instead, He offered her life and gave it freely. *"But whoever drinks the water I give them will never thirst. Indeed, the water I give them will become in them a spring of water welling up to eternal life." The woman said to him, "Sir, give me this water so that I won't get thirsty and have to keep coming here to draw water" (John 4:14–15).*

That must have been some conversation because the woman, despite the five hundred-year-old cultural battle between Samaritans and Jews, felt drawn to Jesus. Believing the Word of Jesus and sensing that He had something great to offer, she asked Him for the living water, and because she asked, she received. Whatever you ask of the Lord, you will receive. This is faith—believing the Word of God to receive what He has already offered to you. This belief gave her transformation of spirit. It filled her with so much joy that she could not contain it; she had to go around and tell everyone of Jesus and what He could offer.

In every man's life exists two types of power: one negative, the other positive. In unexpected times, when we are hit with shocking or troubling news, the negative power has a tendency to take over. This power leads us into depression, anger, and fear. We are not stable during these times, and the heart becomes broken. Darkness enters. Doctors cannot treat these feelings; only the Word of God can heal the broken heart.

Just as the Samaritan woman asked for the water, I also asked for the living water—the Holy Spirit of God. He lovingly gave, and I readily accepted. The interesting thing is that if I had not asked, I would not have received. It is our own responsibility to seek out the Holy Spirit and allow Him to reside within us.

My oncologist noticed this change, and that is why she asked me why I was different from her other patients. As St. Augustine prayed to God many centuries ago: "You have made us for yourself, and our heart is restless until it finds rest in You."

In life, hopelessness, sadness, failure, and sickness exist. It is quite natural. Most people give up and run away, which is easy to do. To do that which is difficult, (i.e., to overcome and move forward) requires the strength of God. The prophet Elijah had success in all that he did; every prophecy he proclaimed came true, and every miracle he performed was done leaving people in amazement and wonder. He had great influence and success over the masses because he operated in the power of Spirit of God. Yet, with all of his success, when Queen Jezebel proclaimed a curse over him, Elijah became filled with fear and ran for his life. He was filled with so much dread that he asked God to take his life. To this man, who desired death, God gave strength by giving him a cake of bread and a jar of water. Elijah took it, ate it, and laid his head down. Again, he was woken up and given food once more because God knew he would need strength for what lay ahead. So he ate and drank and with the strength he gained from that food, he traveled forty days and forty nights until he reached Horeb, the mountain of God. On that mountaintop, God spoke once again to Elijah and told him to do even more for Him. So the man who wanted to end his life moved forward with the Spirit of God and eventually anointed Elisha as a prophet and his successor.

In Job 2:9, his wife advised him to curse God because he had been suffering for so long. She was unable to see hope beyond her present situation. She was a carnal woman who could only understand and accept comfort. Sickness and failure was not acceptable for her kind. But Job's response was, *"You are talking like a foolish woman. Shall we accept good from God, and not trouble?"* Job was a spiritually minded and knew that life was a mix of both good and bad. However, the wife did not have that type of wisdom. The carnal man only wishes for success and health. From this carnal type of thinking, when he comes upon adversity, he curses God, turns to depression, and feels anxiety. Some become very bitter and cannot understand why the sickness must have come to them. They cannot trust God; they do not have the mental capacity. The spiritually minded, however, cannot help but see God's hand over their sickness. The trial is seen as a spiritual gain. There is a hope in the middle of their adversity that God has good in store for them. *"Though I walk in the midst of trouble, you preserve my life. You stretch out your hand against the anger of my foes; with your right hand you save me" (Psalm 138:7).*

Suffering is a part of human life. You have to accept it, but those who grow up in comfort do not have an understanding of suffering. They think that life should be is a bed of roses. Only those who grow up with suffering understand it as a way of life. Believing in God and having faith in His power is the strength of man. The carnal man prides himself in self-achievements. His strength comes from his own ability to be physically strong or mentally smart, so when his physique is weakened or his mental capacity has diminished, he does not know where to turn. He cannot think of God because he has never thought of God before. His pride is low, and he becomes bitter and angry.

I was this carnal man, but through my sickness I came to comprehend a great truth—life is but a breath. What is the benefit of the things I have acquired if I cannot enjoy them? My knowledge is limited. I cannot fully understand the truth in the Word of God. With all of my sins, my pride, and my limitations, I went to my Savior who *is* LOVE and MERCY. In the midst of my sorrow and challenges, instead of growing bitter, I turned to my loving Father with faith and trust. As a result, I received strength as if electricity was flowing through my body. This was the Holy Spirit. The Holy Spirit is a promise. Whoever asks will be filled with the Holy Spirit. Only through faith can you receive it. It does not become ours until we accept and make it our own. By faith—and faith is a gift—we can receive the Holy Spirit, just as it says in scripture: *"By faith we might receive the promise of the Spirit"* (Galatians 3:14).

My fears were gone. My doubt was gone. The next time I went to the doctor, I did not even see myself as a patient. All I could focus on was the hope that lay ahead. Today, I feel like I have the ability to take on the burdens of others even. My transformation was a gift from God.

When we are faced with threats and difficulties in life, it is natural to want to run away. Rather than turning away, if we come to God and take in what He has to give to us, which is the Holy Spirit, then we will have strength to face our trials and do even more than we have done in the past. Although I first lost hope with the news of my cancer, I ate from the Word of God, was given the Holy Spirit, and I was able to be relieved of my depression, fears, and bondages.

Rather than being saddened by others' similar circumstances, I was able to give hope.

My body is dying, this is true. But my spirit is being born again. I have been born again. God has given me a new reason to live. He has given me purpose. My attitude and values have been transformed. My outlook in life has changed. I am a new creation.

Desire the Great Physician above more than you desire the doctors of the world because only He can give you a sound mind. Meditate on the mercies of God, for He will not turn away any who seek Him. Those who desire God will be given a new spirit. Look at your affliction as an opportunity for self-discipline because through it you will receive perseverance and fortitude for future trials, a bright prospect for eternity ahead, and enthusiasm for the life you currently live. All those around you will be able to see this renewed spirit in you.

Promises to Ponder

God created us in His own image and breathed His own breath into our nostrils. We come from a royal family and have the bloodline of God incarnate running through our bodies. But somehow we forget our roots; we live without knowing where we come from. The Bible has many promises from God Himself that encourage us and remind us of our Father, His power, His mercy, and His love for us.

When the Word of God is void in our lives, our minds become cluttered with evil thoughts. How we act will be determined by what we think. Almost every verse is the Bible is a jewel to treasure—you find things like knowledge, understanding, and power. Those who are unable suddenly find ability. Those who are weak find strength. Those who are lonely find a friend in Jesus. Those who hate are filled with love. Those who walk in fear are left with courage.

I hate to remember the time right after I was given news of my cancer. I felt like I was locked up in a cage, and I felt claustrophobic. I was drowning in fear and sadness. I hate to even think like that and I do not want any person to go through that. That was a very sensitive time for me, and it was easy for me to be negatively influenced. I remember a time soon after I was diagnosed when I ate lunch with a co-worker who shared with me his experiences with his aunt who had gone through surgery from breast cancer. He focused on all of the burdensome activities required to care for her. He did not have one positive word to say to me, only negative. After our lunch was over, I felt sick and wished that I had not wasted my time with him, and I longed for someone to tell me that it would be okay.

Death and life are in the words that flow from the tongue.

Those who have a strong faith in God are the ones who can see opportunities in every instance of life, even in sickness. When we dwell on the promises of God, our thinking will shift. Where there is no healing, healing will unexpectedly happen. Where something seemed arduous, it gradually becomes simple.

When you are in sickness, you have an opportunity to humble yourself before God and ASK for help. Many do not ask, thinking they have enough information to heal themselves or that they have enough endurance to stay the course. Some of us humble ourselves and we ASK. Those who ask, receive. As Paul said, *"That is why, for Christ's sake, I delight in weaknesses, in insults, in hardships, in persecutions, in difficulties. For when I am weak, then I am strong" (2 Corinthians 12:10).*

Those who humble themselves receive power from God. God will turn our weaknesses into strength. Moses' weakness was his temper—he became so angry one time that he killed a man. Yet, after he walked with the Lord for some time, the Bible says that he was a humble man—more humble than anyone else on the earth! (Numbers 12:3) How can a murderer have a reputation as the most humble man on earth? Only when God changes him.

For those who think they are unqualified, when they are in the hands of God, they will become qualified. Things like low self-esteem and lack of confidence will no longer exist because God will remove those feelings and replace it with His power. When Gideon was commissioned by God to face his clan's oppressor, Gideon responded by saying that his clan was the weakest and that he was the *least* in his father's house. But God's incredible response was, *"I will be with you, and you will strike down all the Midianites, leaving none alive" (Judges 6:16).* When the angel of God first addressed him, he called him a *"mighty warrior,"* but Gideon did not see himself that way.

God saw him as a mighty man of valor, but Gideon did not!

God saw the strength in Gideon, and He had to push Gideon to believe that he could defeat his enemies.

Today, we are given the words of God, and it is through reading His words that we receive faith in God. Through faith, we receive the Holy Spirit. In the same way that Gideon was given strength, we also will be given strength.

When times are tough and you feel discouraged, I hope you will turn to these verses for a positive answer, for comfort, and for strength:

You say: "It's impossible."
God says: "What is impossible with man is possible with God" (Luke 18:27).

You say: "I'm too tired."
God says: "I will give you rest" (Matthew 11:28).

You say: "Nobody really loves me."
God says: "I love you" (John 3:16, paraphrased).

You say: "I can't go on."
God says: "My grace is sufficient" (2 Corinthians 12:9)

You say: "I can't figure things out."
God says: "I will direct your steps" (Proverbs 3:5–6, paraphrased).

You say: "I can't do it."
God says: "You can do all things" (Philippians 4:13, paraphrased).

You say: "I'm not able."
God says: "I am able" (2 Corinthians 9:8, paraphrased).

You say: "It's not worth it."
God says: "It will be worth it" (Romans 8:28, paraphrased).

You say: "I can't forgive myself."
God says: "I forgive you" (1 John 1:9; Romans 8:1, paraphrased).

You say: "I can't manage."
God says: "I will supply all your needs" (Philippians 4:19, paraphrased).

You say: "I'm afraid."
God says: "I have not given you a spirit of fear" (2 Timothy 1:7, paraphrased).

You say: "I'm always worried and frustrated."
God says: "Cast all your cares on me" (1 Peter 5:7, paraphrased).

You say: "I don't have enough faith."
God says: "I've given everyone a measure of faith" (Romans 12:3, paraphrased).

You say: "I'm not smart enough."
God says: "I give you wisdom" (1 Corinthians 1:30, paraphrased).

You say: "I feel alone."
God says: "Never will I leave you; never will I forsake you" (Hebrews 13:5).

Dolores Karides says it so well. "The greatest peace I've ever known, I found in troubled times, for when I put my trust in God, he eased my troubled mind."[7]

---

[7] Dolores Karides, "Blessed Peace," included in the compilation book of poems *The Joy of Living* by Sara Tarascio, 1986, by Salesian Inspirational Books/Salesian Missions.

To the carnal man, the words of God can seem like a paradox, but in fact, the Word of God is a treasure. It calms the soul. It contains healing. It gives wisdom. It gives strength to the weak. It makes friends of enemies. It makes the impossible possible. God's promises never fail. However, when unbelief and self-sufficiency preside over faith in an Almighty God, the promises may seem difficult to attain, but be patient. Do not give up hope. In God's time, He will enable you to receive His promises.

Seeing brilliant rays amidst dark storm clouds

A diagnosis of breast cancer brings great shock. Women fear breast cancer more than they fear heart disease, even though breast cancer is more treatable and curable. Women tend to go through many emotions at the onset of the diagnosis and throughout treatment. Emotions such as fear, denial, anger, depression, sadness, anxiety, stress, guilt, and loneliness plague the victim's heart. For me, it was numbness—I lost all feeling inside of me and lost my will to live. After the shock set in, I went through anger, guilt, and loneliness. After God worked inside of me, I was gradually transformed.

Two sides exist for every sickness and for every failure. Typically, people tend to focus only on the negative side of these things. When faith is lacking, it is quite natural to be pessimistic. The first stage is denial and anger. Even if someone were to mention the good side to a situation, the sufferer will naturally become annoyed by the positive energy. Even sympathy is not beneficial at this time because offering sympathy only carries that person toward feelings of self-pity.

My feelings were transformed into prayers. My prayers helped me see my pain as part of a divine plan. Because it was from my broken heart, this terrible pain turned me toward a dedication to God.

Getting to Know Myself

Through this hardship, I understood my strengths and my weaknesses. In the same way that dust is seen when sunlight peeks through the window, I was finally able to see the dust (my weaknesses) when my sickness came. Only with my sickness did I reach a point of utter desperation, and I knew that UNLESS I had help from God, I would not be able to press through. It was then that I realized my need for God, and I began to regret greatly that I never really had faith in God. As a child, I was overprotected by my father and as a married woman, I was overprotected by my husband. During my entire life, I was dependent on others. Though my family loved me and did many things for me, they could not take away my fears for me. I had to gird up the strength to persevere during this trial. I had to do it myself; I could not depend on anyone else.

My mother, who is ninety-four years old, is a very spiritual woman who has great passion for the underprivileged. She loves God and her life has been an expression of her love toward God. In fact, my birth was a result of her fervent prayer to God. Although she had five children prior to having me, she desperately wanted another girl. So she fasted and prayed for eight days, specifically for me. God breathed life into my body because of the desire of my mother. I was formed only because I was desired by someone. I never took this seriously. In a house full of children, I never saw my life as precious. I took it for granted. I was very selfish, only desiring to fulfill my needs. I never experienced hardship in my life, either as a child or as a married adult.

God did not create me to be selfish. He created me for a specific purpose, and He filled me with great potential. However, I was blind to my talents. Before my sickness, I had a very narrow mind. As a result, I was always unsatisfied, pessimistic, and filled with complaints. I felt very dull even though I had everything. When God allowed me to experience cancer, I overflowed with emotional distress. I just could not handle the feelings I was experiencing. It was only then that I began to see myself as the negative person I was, and it was only then that I began to see how difficult the lives of others truly were. I began to change and realize that life was not about serving me; rather, it was about serving others. Even cooking for my family was a burden at one time, but now I see it as an absolute joy— to create a beautiful meal for my family whom I love very much.

Perseverance became a characteristic that I greatly wanted to develop. I decided not to complain about my sickness. Instead, I took all of my complaints and weaknesses to God because I wanted to let my children and husband see me in a different light, as a woman who could persevere under trial. Today, I take all my needs to God and He provides me with a peace of mind. When God transformed me from a self-centered person, who was deeply involved in caring for my own self, into a selfless person, who began to see the needs of others as greater than my own, my mind began to expand. Responsibilities that were once burdens have changed into jobs of joy. I saw myself as a mighty warrior and not as a weakened vessel.

Many years prior, I only dreamed of helping other cancer patients, but helping them required certain characteristics to be developed: forgiveness, love, compassion, understanding, patience, and faith. I had none of these traits prior to my cancer, so I was truly not qualified to help other cancer patients. Only after my fight with cancer did I develop these qualities, so my cancer was not meant to bring me harm. It was to qualify me for the task to be a counselor and helper for others going through trials of their own.

"For I know the plans I have for you," declares the LORD, "plans to prosper you and not to harm you, plans to give you hope and a future. Then you will call upon me and come and pray to me, and I will listen to you. You will seek me and find me when you seek me with all your heart" (Jeremiah 29:11–13).

It was my rigid mindset that gave me restlessness. Through my prayers, my disturbed mind became calm. My dependency on money, family, friends, and doctors left. I began, instead, to depend completely on God. THAT was a gift. It also gave me courage.

The Holy Spirit entered into me during my sickness. Following are the blessings of my sickness.

Getting to Know Others

Many times, we do not understand others or take the time to understand them, and I was very much like this. Cancer forced me to change because I had no choice but to hear the testimonies of other survivors and identify with their pain and with their victories. One day during my sickness, I visited a woman who was suffering with cancer. As I began to open up to her, I could tell that she identified with my pain in a way that others simply could not. She also shared with me her anxieties, her freedom from them, and was able to minister to me.

Our surroundings greatly influence us. When we are around positive people, we will eventually see the glass as half full. After my bouts with cancer, when I went to volunteer at a cancer center, I witnessed the dedication of the doctors who were tending to the patients. They were busy, but they were happily busy. It was their determination and hard work that enabled them to be so dedicated to their profession, and I was able to benefit as a result. Because they were knowledgeable in their field, I survived surgery with no infection, received proper treatment with limited side effects, and was prescribed prevention medication that worked right the first time. With patience, they listened to all of the complaints of their patients, and the patients learned to trust them. Their knowledge sharpened my knowledge. As the proverbs says, *"As iron sharpens iron, so one man sharpens another"* *(Proverbs 27:17)*.

It was at this time that I listened to the testimonies of survivors—some even went back to college after their sickness. Reading the biographies of people who endured sickness encouraged me because I kept reading about their unwillingness to give in to the disease. They were survivors who came out on top. Their victories birthed visions inside of me. Rather than focus on my immediate need, I began to fantasize about all the amazing things I would accomplish after my treatment. I developed a strong desire to share my faith. I chose to no longer be a slave of fear or death.

Tolerating cancer and chemotherapy was the toughest thing I have ever had to endure, but once I got to the end, I stood up straight. I was surprised at the stamina that God provided and was even audacious enough to think that I could endure more trials. I believed that I could withstand even more because I came out on top from my first trial. The hardships I went through were for blessings in the future. Through my difficulties, I cultivated inner strength—the strength that God had bestowed upon me but that I only discovered through my trials.

It was during my trials that I understood the power of meditation and what David meant when he said, *"On my bed I remember you; I think of you through the watches of the night" (Psalm 63:6).*

Through meditation, my inner man was strengthened. Through meditation, I began on a journey I had never known before. Through meditation, I received power to do things that previously used to overwhelm me. Life brings with it both blessings and trials. To desire only the blessing is wrong. Jesus will help you through your trials. We are not alone. Jesus Christ enables us through His Holy Spirit to do things that seem impossible, so in our trials we should call upon Him rather than shy away from the task at hand. Hardships are just a part of life. It is easy to give up and run away from it.

No one desires difficulties, but that is not reality. Reality says that difficulties will come. But those who have faith in God understand that this is but a small moment in the vastness of eternity. They talk of their difficulties to God, and He turns their mourning into dancing.

Heart of Patience

Knowing that the proving of your faith worketh patience (James 1:3, ASV).

Patience is not an easy trait to come by. We live in a world where we need everything instantly. Treatments for cancer can take anywhere from six months to over a year, if not more. During this time, there are many sacrifices to make. Your social life has to suffer and the foods you eat have to be limited. It is easy to become depressed, but we must wait patiently for healing. Without complaining, we must wait for healing. For me, it was a time to learn tolerance. I told the Lord all of my troubles, and asked Him to give me strength to handle it all. I became convinced that my sickness was temporary and that it would go away soon. Rather than complaining to my husband, I began to bring all my worries to God, and He provided tolerance. In addition, I received wisdom. I never again saw myself as a disabled sick person.

Be patient, then, brothers and sisters, until the Lord's coming. See how the farmer waits for the land to yield its valuable crop, patiently waiting for the autumn and spring rains (James 5:7).

Just like the farmer who waited patiently, we also must be determined to be patient with the knowledge that God will send His healing. Patience is a fruit of the Holy Spirit. Through my sickness, I received the fruit of patience.

Cancer was my spiritual training ground. It transformed my mind. In order for a student to graduate, he must endure many sleepless nights and long hours of labor to receive his prize. In the same way, we must endure our training ground of sickness. We must learn to accept the temporary problems in life so that we can graduate with honors. Education and intelligence will not give us this gift of patience; only the Holy Spirit can bestow this to us. Those whom God chooses, He trains. Three great men of the Bible—Moses, Joseph, and David—went through intense hardships before they received leadership roles.

Purified Heart

As a cancer survivor, I have to continue my life. I have to continue to cook, clean, tend to my career, fulfill my responsibilities as a mother and grandmother, volunteer with other cancer patients, attend social gatherings, and go to church. I cannot abandon any of these tasks simply because I have cancer. I have to run hard in this race of life. To make it all work, I need mental strength more than I need physical strength. I realize that I need to have a clear mind before my mind can be strengthened. Only then can our emotions be stable. I need control over my mind and my thoughts in order to have a successful life, especially with my sickness. With this control, I can do everything easily without being a burden to others. If there is fear, anger, and other negativity residing in my mind, the remainder of life will be miserable. Perhaps we have received rejection from our co-workers; that's okay. To keep your mind strong, continue meditating on Jesus Christ. This is what I did. I longed only for a pure heart.

The first step in receiving a pure heart is to remove all of the sin from your life. It's called repentance. When God wanted to lead the Israelites to the Promised Land, His first command to them was to remove all the yeast from their home for seven whole days. *"For seven days you are to eat bread made without yeast. On the first day remove the yeast from your houses, for whoever eats anything with yeast in it from the first day through the seventh must be cut off from Israel" (Exodus 12:15).*

Yeast can be compared to sin. We must remove sin from our lives—the sin contained in our thoughts and the sin that comes through our actions. If the thinking is flawed, then the actions will also be flawed. The base of all of this is the heart. If the heart is good, then the thoughts will be pure. If the thoughts are pure, then the fruit (actions) will also be pure. The origin of it all is the heart.

Where does Christ live? In holy places. If our heart is holy, then Christ will abide there. When my sickness came, I was forced to purify my heart. It was only though my sickness that I understood the value of a holy heart. No one could tend to my unholy thoughts; only God could change that. Our duty is to open up our hearts and allow God to live there. God was always knocking at my door, but I only opened it up during my sickness.

Even though God purified my heart during my time of cancer, I desired the purification daily. I saw the value of having a pure heart, and I was addicted to its beauty. Owning a pure heart brought dignity because it removed my shame. It is with this pure heart that I received power to witness to others. It was an incredibly rich experience.

When God resides in our hearts, all darkness is removed. No one will look at us and think that we are diseased people, and we will not see ourselves as diseased people either. Cancer is darkness. But when the light of Christ fills our hearts, feelings of eminence reside. For me, personally, I felt like I was a chosen one. I felt that I had received God's favor. What a great honor it is to receive a pure heart!

Today, when I even mention this God whom I have finally found, I cannot help but feel empowered with the mention of His name. I never cry thinking that I have cancer. However, when I think about this new heart He has given me, I cannot help but cry because I do not understand why He has chosen to give me such an incredible gift. Certainly, I do not deserve it. When I cried out in my pain, God must have felt merciful toward me.

Many of you reading this book may not be a cancer patient, but you may have your own type of darkness. Perhaps your spouse has recently passed; you are suffering with another kind of sickness; you may be depressed; or you are worried about your children.

Rescued from Pharaoh's slavery, the Israelites were placed between a rock and a hard place. In front of them was the looming Red Sea, and from behind they were being pursued by their enemies. Moses encouraged them saying, *"Do not be afraid. Stand firm and you will see the deliverance the LORD will bring you today. The Egyptians you see today you will never see again. The LORD will fight for you; you need only to be still" (Exodus 14:13–14).* Then, from the direction of the Lord, Moses stretched forth his staff and split the Red Sea in half so that the Israelites could pass through on dry ground.

Verses 19 and 20 of Exodus 14 say that the angel of God, who had been traveling in front of Israel's army, withdrew and went behind them. The pillar of cloud also moved from in front and stood behind them, coming between the armies of Egypt and Israel. Throughout the night, the cloud brought darkness to the one side and light to the other side, so neither went near the other all night long.

The Israelites and the Egyptians were in the same place, but God arranged it so that the same cloud brought gloom to one side and illumination to the other side. It's the same in life. For one group, darkness prevails. When does it become dark? When the angel of the Lord moves away from us. But if the angel of the Lord moves in front of us, there is light. When the Lord resides in our hearts, there is radiance, and when the Lord does not reside in our hearts, there is obscurity. Even in our failures, losses, and sicknesses, if God resides in our hearts, we will not fall into misery. Instead, we will remain encouraged and full of hope.

A carnal man may try to depend on others. That is when desolation, anguish, and torment enter into the heart; this is because no human can move the obstacles in our lives. Only the presence of God in our hearts can change our thoughts. Therefore, to make our journeys victorious, we need a purified heart.

"Blessed are the pure in heart, for they will see God" (Matthew 5:8).

Meditating Heart

The word *meditation* comes from the Latin word, *meditari*, which means "to concentrate." Concentration is a very important ability. Only those who have such laser focus can accomplish great things. Meditation is a means to strengthen the spirit. The verses of the Bible are powerful; they offer sacred gifts of peace, comfort, and strength. Psalm 39:3 says, *'My heart grew hot within me. While I meditated, the fire burned; then I spoke with my tongue."* Focusing in such an intense way will set aflame the fire within us. This focus allows us to think of nothing else but God. It forces us to think of His mighty power, and it releases an energy force within us; it causes us to shine. It equips us to take on many challenges. Some verses bring hope. Others bring strength. Still, other verses show how the impossible become possible. Some highlight healing, and other verses bring to light peace. Each verse brings a certain blessing, and focusing or meditating on that verse enables us to pull out that blessing.

No matter what your situation is, the precious Word of God offers a promise and a blessing for it. If we meditate on that verse, we will reap its blessing. For instance, if the situation is a matter of a heavy burden, meditate on the verse that says to bring Him all of your worries because His burden is light and His yolk is easy. Imagine that an incredibly strong person is coming to carry your weight and when you begin to envision this promise, you will begin to reap its blessing.

Everyone desires comfort, and we desire it so much that when discomfort is presented to us, we cannot handle it. This inability can cause us to complain and become depressed. In those situations, we must meditate on Christ. Without even one sin to His name, He carried the rejection and criticism of people. How did Christ take this discomfort? When we begin to dissect how He might have handled this pain, we also recognize how to handle our pain. Our human spirit can cause us to despair. To prevent it, we must meditate on Christ, and we will be able to receive hope and a mind that can take the despair.

If we meditate often, we will also receive strength to forgive. We will receive the character of Christ because we are so focused on

Him. We can repent, we can give thanks, we can remember His many blessings, and we can focus on the fact that He is able to do it. He is able to remove our mountains.

I enjoy going to church and worshiping with others, but I CRAVE meditation because *it* is what gives me joy and strength. Food fattens the body and meditation fattens the soul. It's important to quiet our minds and listen to God. Mediation provides:

1. Meditation provides joy and strength.
2. Meditation provides communion with Jesus.
3. Meditation brings to light the things that are hidden.
4. Mediation also helps us enjoy His presence.
5. Meditation helps us to control our tongues and become better listeners.
6. Meditation helps us to control our thoughts and emotions.

For the word of God is alive and active. Sharper than any double-edged sword, it penetrates even to dividing soul and spirit, joints and marrow; it judges the thoughts and attitudes of the heart (Hebrews 4:12).

Because the Word penetrates our soul, the tired mind receives energy, and the sad mind receives joy. All of our mountains will turn into molehills. We may see a huge burden before us, but when we meditate, we will receive a supernatural mindset—one that is able to handle all that lies before us. This type of wholehearted devotion enables us to take on life's responsibilities. It's in the devotion, not in the intelligence or the education. Devotion also takes sacrifice. Without sacrifice, goals cannot be attained. Sacrifices are hard to endure, but they turn into privileges when we meditate. Christ gave His life to save a sinful person like me. I have also received a mindset to sacrifice my comforts to become more like Christ, but they do not feel like a heavy burden. Rather, it is a joy to serve others now.

"Keep this Book of the Law always on your lips; meditate on it day and night, so that you may be careful to do everything written in it. Then you will be prosperous and successful" (Joshua 1:8).

Joshua commanded the people to meditate on the Word of God so that they could be prosperous. In the same way, we also should meditate so that we can become successful.

Forgiving Heart

Stress comes from built up guilt, inability to forgive, and lack of trust in God. Stress is relieved when you accept the forgiveness of God. When we approach a holy God, we are able to see our filthiness. When we remove pride from our hearts and approach the throne of God, He bestows mercy, and we will be able to forget all the things we did in our past.

"I, even I, am he who blots out your transgressions, for my own sake, and remembers your sins no more" (Isaiah 43:25).

When we can believe wholeheartedly in this promise of forgiveness, then our old stress-filled heart will be replaced with a new stress-free heart. God's forgiveness was not given because of our doing; rather, it is a free gift from Him. God expects us to forgive others in the same way He forgave us. The common man finds it difficult to forgive. Even one wrong word makes him sensitive. As a result, he fights for no reason. This increases stress. Instead, we should be able to overlook another person's actions, forgive that person, and consider him unaware of his dealings with us. Remember, they may not walk with the Holy Spirit. Rather than finding vengeance with that person, we should pray for him to receive the power of the Holy Spirit in the same way that we received it.

It takes grace to pray for someone who is hurting you; it is easy to consider revenge. Grace is a gift of the Holy Spirit, and it brings incredible joy. Isn't this how Christ treated His enemies? While hanging on the cross, beaten, He never once argued back, but rather He prayed *"Father, forgive them, for they do not know what they are doing" (Luke 23:34).* When we desire to come into this type of grace, then He will fulfill it. It is the desire that will bring it to us.

There is a story in the Bible of David and Saul. Saul hunted David for a long part of his life, but when David had the opportunity to kill Saul, he withdrew and feared God. David saw Saul sleeping

183

in a cave and could have taken his life. Instead, he cut off a piece of Saul's garment to prove to Saul his grace. When Saul found out, he said to David, *"You are more righteous than I," he said. "You have treated me well, but I have treated you badly. You have just now told me about the good you did to me; the Lord delivered me into your hands, but you did not kill me. When a man finds his enemy, does he let him get away unharmed? May the Lord reward you well for the way you treated me today. I know that you will surely be king and that the kingdom of Israel will be established in your hands"* (1 Samuel 24:17–20).

We live freely today because our God has given us incredible forgiveness. God expects us to forgive others in the same way He forgave us. We are obliged. When Peter asked Jesus if he should forgive up to seven times, Jesus replied, "I do not say to you, up to seven times, but up to seventy times seven" (Matthew 18:22, NASB).

The kingdom of heaven is likened to a king who wanted to settle accounts with his servants. One man owed ten thousand bags of gold and did not have the means to pay off his debt. The king told him to sell all that he had, including his wife and children, so that he could earn enough to pay back the king. This brought great difficulty to him. From the pain that he felt deep within his heart, he fell down before the king and begged him to forgive him his debt. The king took pity on him, and let him go debt free.

The man who received forgiveness did the exact opposite. After receiving forgiveness from the king, he went on his way. On the road, he ran into a man who owed him a hundred silver coins. Forgetting all the mercy and grace that had just been bestowed on him, he grabbed the neck of the man who owed him money. Even though this servant begged for mercy, he refused and threw him into prison instead.

Seeing this, his fellow servants, feeling badly, approached the king and told him about what transpired. The king became angry and demanded to know why he could not offer the same type of mercy toward his servant that the king had offered to him. He did not have an answer, so the king handed him over to the jailers to be tortured.

Jesus says that if we don't forgive others, then God the Father will do the same to us. If we do not have the grace to forgive, we will be tortured by our own guilt. If we look at the past, we can easily see that it is solely by the grace of God that we have lived this far. All of the blessings we have today are because of a forgiving Father. Always keep in mind that we have received forgiveness from many around us—parents, teachers, co-workers, and friends. Therefore, we are indebted to offer forgiveness to others; otherwise, we are at risk of eluding the forgiveness of God.

Heart of Gratitude

Before my cancer, if I ever received anything like a job, an education, a home, or my good health, I just went on my way thinking that it was because of my hard work. Even though I worked in a children's hospital and witnessed children who were born with serious birth defects, I never thought to give thanks to God for my own health. I just took for granted all that I was blessed with. Only after I went through cancer did I really appreciate my health. When my health was taken away from me, it came as such a shock. When I had nothing but good health, I did not understand its value, but when it was taken away from me, I cherished it. Only when what we have is stripped away do we understand its importance.

Most of us tend to have a grumbling character, always looking after things we do not have rather than appreciating what we do have. When the Israelites were wandering through the desert, they were fed by God every day with fresh manna from heaven and fresh water from the rocks. Rather than being grateful for all the things that He had given to them, they complained about not having meat to eat. So God, with fury in His heart, brought an abundance of quail for them to eat. While they put the meat between their teeth and before they could consume it, He brought a plague and killed all those who had craved meat.

This is how it is in our lives. If we always complain and grumble about what we do not have and do not pause to thank God for what we *do* have, we will live life with no satisfaction. If we offer help to someone and they give thanks, imagine the satisfaction we receive from their gratefulness. In fact, it encourages us to give them more.

Luke 17 tells the story of the ten lepers who healed when Jesus was on His way to Jerusalem. Only one came back and fell at the feet of Jesus and gave thanks—he was a Samaritan and not a Jew. Jesus asked, *"Were not all ten cleansed? Where are the other nine? Has no one returned to give praise to God except this foreigner?" (Luke 17:17–18).* So you see that Jesus expects us to give thanks. When we get healing or receive any blessing from God, we should be thankful to God. When we have a heart of thanks, we also receive more of a blessing. It is a heart that honors God, and this brings satisfaction to our souls.

Every morning, we should be thankful that God has given us another day. I did not used to have this kind of gratefulness, but today I wake up with joy, thankful that He has given me a second chance at life. This is such a great feeling, this feeling of thankfulness.

Even if we have ninety-nine things to be thankful for and one thing that we are worried about, we will grumble about the one thing. We need to train up our mind to count our blessings. When we see our blessings rather than our grumblings, joy abounds and complaints cease.

Give thanks in all circumstances; for this is God's will for you in Christ Jesus (1 Thessalonians 5:18).

Joyful Heart

Paul, in the book of Philippians, says to rejoice always. How can you do that? When we have everything, we are happy. With successes come happiness and with failures come sorrow. But life is not filled with only successes; there is a fair share of failures as well. Joy comes from the heart. Happiness is found in successes, but joy comes from within. How can we attain joy? Only we control what is poured into our hearts; we have authority over what fills our minds. During our failures and sicknesses, when we fill our hearts with the Word of God rather than the trial, we live in the presence of God Himself. When the verses reign in our hearts, it begins to rule our thoughts.

And I heard a loud voice from the throne saying, "Look! God's dwelling place is now among the people, and he will dwell with them. They will be his people, and God himself will be with them and be their God. He will wipe every tear from their eyes. There will be no more death' or mourning or crying or pain, for the old order of things has passed away" (Revelation 21:3–4).

The presence of God brings fullness of joy.

Even in sickness.

We may cry, but we will not be depressed. When the words of God reside in our hearts, we begin to dream. We think of hopeful things—that the sickness will get better and that even in death, we will live forever. The joy of the Lord brings strength because even in sickness, we live in the presence of Almighty God! Our thinking is transformed, and we begin to understand that it is best to live with faith. We gain a deep understanding of the wisdom of walking close with the Lord.

To live a life filled with joy, the Word of God must always abide in our hearts. Every morning, during my meditation time, I ask the Lord not to leave me. If my mind is weak, I can face nothing else in the day. Before I eat my breakfast, I nourish my soul. When I am filled with His divine presence, others witness the joy in my heart. Many people have success in the world, but they do not have joy. Yet, everyone desires joy. No one likes to be miserable.

There is a story in the Bible that tells of the seventy-two men that Jesus sent out to minister in the town. He gave them the power of the Holy Spirit so that they were able to heal sicknesses and cast out demons in His name. The seventy-two men rejoiced because of their newfound power and happily proclaimed it to Jesus, but Jesus responded, *"do not rejoice that the spirits submit to you, but rejoice that your names are written in heaven" (Luke 10:1–20).*

Through my sickness, I was given a chance to think about heaven and that my name was written in the Book of Life. After cancer, I always think about the gift that God has given to me; I no longer worry about the sickness—that fear has been completely wiped clean. Now, for the rest of my life, I will live by walking right with the Lord; I no longer fear sickness or trial. I live with the grace of God, which brings great power. It enables me to carry great responsibilities, to forgive all of my enemies, and to live with incredible joy. Great joy is found in the recesses of my heart because that is where the Word of God resides.

"You make known to me the path of life; you will fill me with joy in your presence, with eternal pleasures at your right hand" (Psalm 16:11).

Hopeful Heart

Hope is what sustains us. For some, sickness brings with it thoughts of depression—almost as if the end of your life has arrived. At first, the idea of life beyond sickness is difficult to grasp. When we dwell in this bleak mindset, even the treatment will not be effective. Essentially, if we do not have hope, we give up. It is important to dream of things that we can do after our healing. It is important to visualize also. We must "see" the things that we will do after our healing.

When Lazarus died, Jesus said that his sickness would not end in death, but rather it would glorify the Son of God (John11:4). In the same way, my sickness would not end in death. Rather, I was being used as a vessel to bring glory to the Son of God. This verse brought great hope.

One day, while visiting India, I stayed for two months at my brother and sister-in-law's house in India—Alex and Susan. While there, we shared stories, cooked together, and did some gardening, a hobby that I really take pleasure in. Each day, I would share my faith that I received through my sickness. They saw this as a great gift—to be able to hear of my trials and victories and the faith that I attained through it all. We thoroughly enjoyed ourselves. After our departure back to the States, Susan called me one day and said that she had kept up with the gardening in hopes that I would go back and stay with them again.

Jesus tells us in John 14:3, *"And if I go and prepare a place for you, I will come back and take you to be with me that you also may be where I am."* The Son of the Most High God came down from His heavenly throne to dwell with sinful man and when He left, He committed to us His Holy Spirit and went to prepare a place for us. Even when we leave this earth, there is a place that has been prepared for us in heaven. We must be sure of this.

A Christian should have hope. There is hope that a home has

been prepared for us. In heaven, there are many mansions prepared for us. Do not focus on the troubles of this world; focus instead on the victory of Jesus. Believing in a God who is almighty and all powerful is what gives us hope. Our sicknesses will be healed and our sins will be forgiven. This brings hope. This God gives to us salvation, which also brings hope.

Hope is not received through any merit of our own. No, it is received through the blood of Christ. God has brought us to salvation. We must narrow our thoughts to the promises of God. When we focus on an eternity in heaven, we receive hope. At an unexpected time when I was told that I was a cancer patient, hope was stripped away from me. Living without hope is dreadful. A young lady told me about her mother who was diagnosed with cancer and was healed. However, the news of the cancer brought such hopelessness to the mother that she died, not because of the disease, but because of a deep-rooted depression, which stemmed from a feeling of hopelessness. Cancer of the body is treatable; however, the disease of the mind cannot be treated by a physician. God, however, will give both physical and mental healing. Just believe. Psalm 55:4–8 says:

> [4] "My heart is in anguish within me;
> the terrors of death have fallen on me.
> [5] Fear and trembling have beset me;
> horror has overwhelmed me.
> [6] I said, "Oh, that I had the wings of a dove!
> I would fly away and be at rest.
> [7] I would flee far away
> and stay in the desert;
> [8] I would hurry to my place of shelter,
> far from the tempest and storm."

This world is full of sorrow and death; it comes to all without discrimination. When it comes, do not give up and do not get discouraged. As David said, hurry to your place of shelter—to God—who is far from the tempest and storm.

Complaints Turned to Praises

The realization of the brevity of life brings wisdom. It is this understanding that can motivate us to move from complacency to zealousness. In my own life, I never experienced great sickness, and I never thought much about death. My life was just one breath after another, with no thought of eternity ahead and certainly no thought of its finality. Facing difficulties, whether small or great, brought nothing but complaints from my lips. My tolerance level was low because I desired nothing more than to sit in the seat of comfort. My sickness was a wake-up call. God threw me out of my comfort zone to turn my complaints into praises. Prior to this time, I had never maximized my talents and never realized my potential. I craved comfort over hard work. Even something as simple as cooking used to be a burden, and I would approach it with a heavy heart. Today, God has changed my attitude. Rather than looking at cooking as a chore, I see it as an opportunity to thank God for my two arms and for the finances we have to purchase the food we are able to cook. Because of my changed heart (now filled with gratitude), my cooking has improved!

"Develop an attitude of gratitude, and give thanks for everything that happens to you, knowing that every step forward is a step toward achieving something bigger and better than your current situation." —Brian Tracy[8]

Learn to Meditate

We live in this world with lots of challenges. The Bible never promised a life without challenges. The world is filled with difficulties, but the One who overcame the troubles remains with us. Faith in the One who is able to carry these burdens enables us to overcome also. Prior to my faith in God, I trusted in man, but those who I had depended on could not even handle their own struggles. They could not separate me from my negative thoughts. No one person could carry my heart's pain or physical sickness.

The outer man was shaken, so there was no choice but to fortify the inner man. The race we run is to nourish our outer man. With or without our knowledge, our inner man is left starving and

[8] Brian Tracy, author speaker, http://briantracy.com/

no effort is put into building him up. Greater than the pain of the physical is the pain of the soul. Doctors can treat the body's pain; however, doctors cannot treat the soul. Only the Word of God can minister to the inner man, the soul.

Before my sickness, I was satisfied with church worship, my family prayer, and my personal prayer life. After my sickness, I came to understand that those aspects of worship were not enough for me, so I gave myself to reading the Word of God and meditating. I focused on the Word and repeated it over and over so that I came to believe it with all of my heart. In doing so, I was able to trust that the promise was for me. Thus, my heart was comforted, encouraged, and rejuvenated. This became a practice for me. I would wake up at 4:30 in the morning when all was quiet and no one was around in order to meditate on the incredible Word of God. I found so much power in His Word. This practice brought me peace of mind, hope, and strength; anxiety no longer had its control over me.

The Bible has many stories of the masses reaching out to Jesus for healing. I would visualize this occurrence in my head. Just like the lady who had been bleeding for twelve years dared to conceive the notion that Jesus would give her healing, I also was provoked to believe that this same Jesus could possibly grant me healing. Just like the lady approached him with a pure heart, I would also need to draw near to Him with a pure heart. So I did. In the wee hours of the morning, I sat before my Father's feet and thanked Him for all that He had given to me, and I nourished myself with His promises. Before I ate to fill my belly, I meditated to fill my soul.

When your words came, I ate them; they were my joy and my heart's delight" (Jeremiah 15:16).

Meditating (that is, repeating) the Word of God is the formula to receiving power. Meditating enables us to build up our faith. Just like pouring cold water into a bowl filled with hot water will cool it down, pouring the Word of God into our tempered souls cools it down. Just like the heat of the water is slowly dissipated, the heat of our emotions, anxieties, sorrows, and sicknesses will be consumed and dissolved by the Holy Spirit. He leaves us, then, with good thoughts— thoughts that empower us and help us to see the might of God.

Powerful Heart

Going through this experience with cancer has given me new eyes and a new heart. It has shown me that I am not the only one suffering. No, in fact there are many who are in my shoes. My mission in life has become to strengthen them. This takes courage, which is given to us by God without any discrimination. It is dependent only on a willing heart, and thank God I had a willing heart. This willing heart brought me to my knees and allowed me to accept the incredible power of the Holy Spirit. Sometimes your mind (your own enemy) will try to convince you that you cannot do anything. Sometimes your visitors will sympathize and cry with hopelessness. Don't believe these lies. You are chosen. God will heal you. He is able. I believe that God was purifying me and refining me through my trial. He was softening my heart. God now dwells permanently in my heart, and He whispers His promises to me moment by moment. The Word resides in my heart continuously.

The great judge, Samson, was given extraordinary strength by God, but he callously disobeyed and that strength was taken away. It is almost as if he had taken for granted all the blessings of God. He did not need to call out to Him for anything because God had created him as a powerful being. Interestingly, it was in the midst of his utter fragility—when he was left blind and weak—that he actually asked God to give to him what he had once lost. It was in his moment of final weakness that he was convicted enough to call upon His maker for power. It was only then that the zenith of his power was realized.

Then Samson prayed to the LORD, "Sovereign LORD, remember me. Please, God, strengthen me just once more, and let me with one blow get revenge on the Philistines for my two eyes." . . . Then he pushed with all his might, and down came the temple on the rulers and all the people in it. Thus he killed many more when he died than while he lived (Judges 16:28, 30).

Samson received a double portion of strength at the end of his life, so much so that he was able to affect twice as many people with it than he had during the entire course of his life. In the same way that Samson received renewed power when he was at his weakest, I also received an increased share of strength during my most vulnerable time. I no longer wanted to remain in hopelessness, fear of death, and fear of others, so I took the brewing force of His spirit and flung away my crippling handicaps.

Because of His mercy, I was freely given the Holy Spirit. For my beloved readers, please know that He is knocking at your heart also; open up your heart for Him so that He can live in your heart, deliver you from bondage (negative thoughts), and give you the courage to weather your trials.

The truth will set you free.

Physical exercise strengthens muscles. Likewise, life's afflictions build stamina because the struggles open our eyes to our finiteness, enabling us to trust in God. As a result, trials really become a stepping-stone to promotion, through which we find the path to our divine destinies.

Payday

Paychecks are typically given weekly, bi-weekly, or monthly. Everyone who receives a check is happy to get paid for his work. Life is similar to this. While we live, there are many things we are required to do. After that, we have to face death. As I learned, death for the believer is indeed a time of celebration.

Only when I first learned of my cancer did I begin to consider death as a reality. Prior to that, I really never gave it much thought. Fear is often a result of ignorance; not fully understanding a matter can bring great fear in the situation. I was afraid of death because I did not know much about it. In the Word of God, death is discussed quite frequently, and often in correlation with hope, joy, and freedom, but I did not pay attention to it. I did not give much thought to it, so I did not have faith that with death came great joy.

During my time of chemo and surgery, I did not dare think about death. It was only after I went through all of my treatment that I began to journey through the Bible on the topic of death. The apostle Paul's thoughts, in particular, influenced me. Philippians 1:21 says, *"For to me, to live is Christ and to die is gain."* 1 Corinthians 15:55 says, *"Where, O death, is your victory? Where, O death, is your sting?"*

As I meditated on these types of verses, I began to realize that Paul was a human just like me. He even fought against Christianity at one time in his life. But once he became a new creation, he began to be bold in his thoughts about death. I asked God to give me this new way of thinking because death is inevitable. Death will affect the president, the king, the pope, the limo driver, the tax collector, the poor, and the rich. No one is discriminated against, and no one knows when his time will be up. The person who faces death faces it by himself. No one can face it with him—not his wife, not his children, and not his pets. The only One who will be there is Jesus Christ Himself. Jesus leaves us with a promise in John 14 that He is going away to prepare a place for us. Believe in Jesus Christ. Just believe. He is going to His Father's house to prepare rooms for us.

I used to read these verses with my worldly intelligence and was not able to grasp the meaning. Today, I read this with my spirit so I believe it deeply. I had told God to give me the mind of a three-year-old, and He has given me this wonderful gift. I can believe these Words of His with a simple faith.

As Paul said: *"to live is Christ and to die is gain" (Philippians 1:21).* Again, in Revelation 14:13 it says, *"Blessed are the dead who die in the Lord from now on." "Yes," says the Spirit, "they will rest from their labor, for their deeds will follow them."* Those who die in Christ are blessed, but in order to die in Christ, we must first live in Christ.

In the book of Numbers, Balaam was offered a large sum of money by King Balaak to curse the Israelites. King Balaak was afraid of the growing number of Israelites, so he wanted Balaam to curse them. However, God had specifically told Balaam not to say anything unless He Himself had put the words in Balaam's mouth. For the most part, Balaam was obedient to God. He wanted desperately to die the death of a righteous man. He said, *"Let me die the death of the righteous, and may my final end be like theirs!" (Numbers 23:10).* However, after King Balaak tempted him over and over with all the kingdoms that could be his and all the power that he could attain, Balaam found a way to bring curses on the Israelites without defiling himself publicly. He counseled the Moabite king to offer the Moabite women to the Israelite men in whoredom. When these vile acts were committed, Israel brought curses upon themselves. *"They were the ones who followed Balaam's advice and enticed the Israelites to be unfaithful to the LORD in the Peor incident, so that a plague struck the LORD'S people" (Numbers 31:16).*

Even though Balaam desired to die as a righteous man, his wish did not come true. Numbers 31:8 says, *"They also killed Balaam son of Beor with the sword."*

Most people set noble goals for themselves, but many cannot reach their goals. Balaam wanted to die the death of a righteous man, but he could not attain it. Similarly, the Christian life is a race. The apostle Paul compares life to a race; our focus should always be on the goal. We should not worry about who is in front of us, beside us, or behind us. Just as the audience cheers on the runner, we also need cheerleaders to encourage us through. The runner is focused solely on the finish line.

Success in life also requires our focus to be on the finish line. Many people, however, turn back and look at what is behind and what the past had to offer, even though it can never be regained. But what God's love allows us to do is forget what was left behind and focus on what's ahead. The race of life is not without obstacles and certainly not without temptations. As we allow ourselves to be tempted, we allow ourselves to veer off track and remove our eyes from the goal. Those who keep their eyes focused on the past cannot move forward with ease. They Lve with lots of regret and approach things with a heaviness.

To reach the finish line, it is more important for our minds to be strong than for our bodies to be strong; otherwise, we will easily be sidetracked. The mind is the rudder that steers the ship. It is the engine that runs the car. It is the determination and will power of a person's mind that allows him or her to move to a higher level of success in life. It is very important for the cancer patient to mold and grow a powerful mind because while the doctor can remove the physical infirmity, he cannot do anything with the will or determination of a man's mind.

No one enjoys failure. Everyone desires to be a victor. But to be a victor, we must be our own disciplinarians. In every marathon, runners prepare themselves in a certain way; they avoid solid foods, they keep themselves hydrated, and they try to maintain a steady pace while running. All runners must have crossed the finish line by a certain time.

Life also has a time limit. Some are given fifty years, some sixty, and some eighty. Some are even blessed to live into their hundreds! To prepare for the end, we must keep our souls hydrated with the Word of God. Otherwise, the soul will cry on the inside, which can lead to depression and lack of satisfaction in life. Only God's Word can satisfy the soul. Each person must seek this out himself. He has to recognize his soul's need for the Word of God and then he must ask God to fill that void. When he asks, God gives. When God gives, satisfaction comes, forgiveness is brought, and deep joy is experienced.

The Christian life is not a life of comfort. When the Israelites were freed from Egypt, they had a goal ahead to reach the Promised Land. They did not go through comfort to reach their goal. There were deserts, raging waters, lack of food and water, and discouraging words. They went through rebellion and desired to turn back to their land of bondage. Only Caleb and Joshua held the faith, so only they were able to see the Promised Land. The Israelites had to overcome many, many difficulties and trials to reach the Promised Land, and we too must face many, many difficulties to reach our goals.

Rather than getting discouraged with these misfortunes, it is important to keep our eyes on the goal and run the race with vigor. In the end, we will receive a crown. Those who cross the finish line will receive the promises of God as it says in scripture:

Revelation 2:7 says, *"To the one who is victorious, I will give the right to eat from the tree of life, which is in the paradise of God."*

Revelation 2:17 says, *"To the one who is victorious, I will give some of the hidden manna. I will also give that person a white stone with a new name written on it, known only to the one who receives it."*

Revelation 2:26 says, *"To the one who is victorious and does my will to the end, I will give authority over the nations."*

Revelation 3:5 says, *"The one who is victorious will, like them, be dressed in white. I will never blot out the name of that person from the book of life, but will acknowledge that name before my Father and his angels."*

Revelation 3:12 says, *"The one who is victorious I will make a pillar in the temple of my God. Never again will they leave it. I will write on them the name of my God and the name of the city of my God, the new Jerusalem, which is coming down out of heaven from my God; and I will also write on them my new name."*

Revelation 3:21 says, *"To the one who is victorious, I will give the right to sit with me on my throne, just as I was victorious and sat down with my Father on his throne."*

These are all of God's promises. God's promises stand true; they are not like the promises of man. Everything God promises will come to pass. We must run our race well. Sickness, challenges, adversities, and the like will stand in the way, but we must not lose focus. Mary and Martha worried about who would move the stone to the entrance of Jesus' tomb, but when they arrived, the angels had already moved it for them. In the same way, I know that all of my large stones will be moved by God. I will receive super natural strength to finish my race. I will not allow anything to distract me from the goal. I spend every morning in meditation. I confess all of my weaknesses to my strong and able God. A divine guidance from the inside leads me on. God has a crown stored away for me because I believe *"I have fought the good fight, I have finished the race, I have kept the faith"* (2 Timothy 4:6).

Our race in life is to obtain that crown. When we keep our eyes on that crown, the worries of the world melt away. The hardships in life become small compared to the crown of life waiting for us. When I committed myself to God, He gave me eternal life in heaven. It is a gift that I do not deserve. I often ask God what I have done to deserve this wonderful gift. Nothing. But He has still given me peace, hope, and joy. I do not know how much longer I have to live. One thing I do know—tribulation will come. But let it come because I have an authority living in me that enables me to overcome. Tears and heartache will come to every life, yet when our good Lord dwells with us, He will wipe away those tears and provide comfort. Believing in the Word of God is what gives hope because eternity has been promised to us. Revelation 21:3 says, "And I heard a loud voice from the throne saying, 'Look! God's dwelling place is now among the people, and he will dwell with them. They will be his people, and God himself will be with them and be their God.'" Even though this is a revelation of the new earth and the new heaven, this is what has happened to me. God took His dwelling in me and because of that, I received hope and was set free from the fear of death. I believe that God dwells with me here on this earth, and when I die, I will dwell with God in heaven. I do not claim any of this from my own merit; rather, I just believe this is the promise of God. Only those who believe that God dwells within are those who will receive hope, salvation, and an eternity with Him.

Revelation 22:17 says, "The Spirit and the bride say, 'Come!' And let the one who hears say, 'Come!' Let the one who is thirsty come; and let the one who wishes take the free gift of the water of life." Through the experience of my cancer, I experienced a thirst for eternity—for the water of life. When I desired it, through God's mercy, He gave me the promise of eternity. Of all the good that I have received, this is the most precious blessing of my breast cancer—the gift of eternal life in heaven.

Run the race of life with the crown in mind because God wants you to spend eternity with Him. There is no suffering in heaven, so look with hope toward that promise in the midst of your own afflictions. Learn how to find hope despite the disappointments; it is the only way to achieve complete and total healing and receive peace.

Epilogue

$\mathcal{I}$never thought I would write this book. In order to write this book, God allowed me to go through a dark tunnel (breast cancer). In the midst of my pain, I turned to Jesus Christ in faith and trust. He was the only One who could control my emotions and my negative thoughts. Man is mortal, and he will change. But the Word of God never changes. Today, I think that pain was worth it. Through that pain and true repentance, my heart was purified. I have no more fear and no more anxiety; instead, I received the huge gift of SALVATION. When I received this free gift through the love and mercy of God, I thought about others who were going through the same situation as I did, and I wanted to help. As I thought about others, He blessed me with twice as much as I had before.

First, my heavenly Father blessed me with His powerful words that sustain the weary. When these powerful words came to my heart, I had the strength to write this book. Jesus Christ filled me with His Holy Spirit to encourage the timid and help the weak.

And second, my daughter, Benji, recently took a test that checks for hereditary cancer genes and found that her results were negative; she did not inherit the gene that would cause cancer! Praise God!

I know God can do all things.

Appendix:
What you need to know about breast cancer[9]

As a breast cancer survivor, I believe healing only comes if the mind, spirit, soul, and body are touched equally. Only God can provide that healing. When we yearn for His grace, the yearning produces a faith that is planted firmly in God. For the body to heal, we need the proper knowledge of cancer and how to best treat the symptoms and disease. Below is an excerpt from the National Cancer Institute, which will elaborate on the disease, treatment options, types of tests, and how to diagnose. I hope this information blesses you. Thank you to the National Cancer Institute for making this freely available for use.

Cancer Cells

Cancer begins in cells, the building blocks that make up tissues. Tissues make up the breasts and other parts of the body.

Normal cells grow and divide to form new cells as the body needs them. When normal cells grow old or get damaged, they die, and new cells take their place.

Sometimes, this process goes wrong. New cells form when the body doesn't need them, and old or damaged cells don't die as they should. The buildup of extra cells often forms a mass of tissue called a lump, growth, or tumor.

[9] The National Cancer Institute, "What You Need to Know about Cancer," http://www.cancer.gov/cancertopics/wyntk/breast (posted 10/15/2009). This text may be reproduced or reused freely.

Tumors in the breast can be benign (not cancer) or malignant (cancer). Benign tumors are not as harmful as malignant tumors:

Benign Tumors

- are rarely a threat to life
- can be removed and usually don't grow back
- don't invade the tissues around them
- don't spread to other parts of the body

Malignant Tumors

- may be a threat to life
- often can be removed but sometimes grow back
- can invade and damage nearby organs and tissues (such as the chest wall)
- can spread to other parts of the body

Breast cancer cells can spread by breaking away from the original tumor. They enter blood vessels or lymph vessels, which branch into all the tissues of the body. The cancer cells may be found in lymph nodes near the breast. The cancer cells may attach to other tissues and grow to form new tumors that may damage those tissues.

The spread of cancer is called metastasis.

Symptoms

Early breast cancer usually doesn't cause symptoms. But as the tumor grows, it can change how the breast looks or feels. The common changes include:

- A lump or thickening in or near the breast or in the underarm area
- A change in the size or shape of the breast
- Dimpling or puckering in the skin of the breast
- A nipple turned inward into the breast
- Discharge (fluid) from the nipple, especially if it's bloody

- Scaly, red, or swollen skin on the breast, nipple, or areola (the dark area of skin at the center of the breast). The skin may have ridges or pitting so that it looks like the skin of an orange.

Detection and Diagnosis

Your doctor can check for breast cancer before you have any symptoms. During an office visit, your doctor will ask about your personal and family medical history. You'll have a physical exam. Your doctor may order one or more imaging tests, such as a mammogram.

Doctors recommend that women have regular clinical breast exams and mammograms to find breast cancer early. Treatment is more likely to work well when breast cancer is detected early.

Clinical Breast Exam

During a clinical breast exam, your health care provider checks your breasts. You may be asked to raise your arms over your head, let them hang by your sides, or press your hands against your hips.

Mammogram

A mammogram is an x-ray picture of tissues inside the breast. Mammograms can often show a breast lump before it can be felt. They also can show a cluster of tiny specks of calcium. These specks are called microcalcifications. Lumps or specks can be from cancer, precancerous cells, or other conditions. Further tests are needed to find out if abnormal cells are present.

Before they have symptoms, women should get regular screening mammograms to detect breast cancer early:

- Women in their 40s and older should have mammograms every 1 or 2 years.
- Women who are younger than 40 and have risk factors for breast cancer should ask their health care provider whether to have mammograms and how often to have them.

If the mammogram shows an abnormal area of the breast, your doctor may order clearer, more detailed images of that area. Doctors use diagnostic mammograms to learn more about unusual breast changes, such as a lump, pain, thickening, nipple discharge, or change in breast size or shape. Diagnostic mammograms may focus on a specific area of the breast. They may involve special techniques and more views than screening mammograms.

Other Imaging Tests

If an abnormal area is found during a clinical breast exam or with a mammogram, the doctor may order other imaging tests:

- **Ultrasound**: A woman with a lump or other breast change may have an ultrasound test. An ultrasound device sends out sound waves that people can't hear. The sound waves bounce off breast tissues. A computer uses the echoes to create a picture. The picture may show whether a lump is solid, filled with fluid (a cyst), or a mixture of both. Cysts usually are not cancer. But a solid lump may be cancer.
- **MRI:** MRI uses a powerful magnet linked to a computer. It makes detailed pictures of breast tissue. These pictures can show the difference between normal and diseased tissue.

Biopsy

A biopsy is the removal of tissue to look for cancer cells. A biopsy is the only way to tell for sure if cancer is present.

Staging

If the biopsy shows that you have breast cancer, your doctor needs to learn the extent (stage) of the disease to help you choose the best treatment. The stage is based on the size of the cancer, whether the cancer has invaded nearby tissues, and whether the cancer has spread to other parts of the body.

- **Bone scan:** The doctor injects a small amount of a radioactive substance into a blood vessel. It travels through the bloodstream and collects in the bones. A machine called a scanner detects and measures the radiation. The scanner makes pictures of the bones. The pictures may show cancer that has spread to the bones.
- **CT scan:** Doctors sometimes use CT scans to look for breast cancer that has spread to the liver or lungs. An x-ray machine linked to a computer takes a series of detailed pictures of your chest or abdomen. You may receive contrast material by injection into a blood vessel in your arm or hand. The contrast material makes abnormal areas easier to see.
- **Lymph node biopsy:** The stage often is not known until after surgery to remove the tumor in your breast and one or more lymph nodes under your arm. Surgeons use a method called sentinel lymph node biopsy to remove the lymph node most likely to have breast cancer cells. The surgeon injects a blue dye, a radioactive substance, or both near the breast tumor. Or the surgeon may inject a radioactive substance under the nipple. The surgeon then uses a scanner to find the sentinel lymph node containing the radioactive substance or looks for the lymph node stained with dye. The sentinel node is removed and checked for cancer cells. Cancer cells may appear first in the sentinel node before spreading to other lymph nodes and other places in the body.

These tests can show whether the cancer has spread and, if so, to what parts of your body. When breast cancer spreads, cancer cells are often found in lymph nodes under the arm (axillary lymph nodes). Also, breast cancer can spread to almost any other part of the body, such as the bones, liver, lungs, and brain.

When breast cancer spreads from its original place to another part of the body, the new tumor has the same kind of abnormal cells and the same name as the primary (original) tumor. For example, if breast cancer spreads to the bones, the cancer cells in the bones are actually breast cancer cells. The disease is metastatic breast cancer, not bone cancer. For that reason, it is treated as breast cancer, not bone cancer. Doctors call the new tumor "distant" or metastatic disease.

These are the stages of breast cancer:

- **Stage 0** is sometimes used to describe abnormal cells that are not invasive cancer. For example, Stage 0 is used for ductal carcinoma in situ (DCIS). DCIS is diagnosed when abnormal cells are in the lining of a breast duct, but the abnormal cells have not invaded nearby breast tissue or spread outside the duct. Although many doctors don't consider DCIS to be cancer, DCIS sometimes becomes invasive breast cancer if not treated.

- **Stage I** is an early stage of invasive breast cancer. Cancer cells have invaded breast tissue beyond where the cancer started, but the cells have not spread beyond the breast. The tumor is no more than 2 centimeters (three-quarters of an inch) across.

- **Stage II** is one of the following:

  o The tumor is no more than 2 centimeters (three-quarters of an inch) across. The cancer has spread to the lymph nodes under the arm.

  o The tumor is between 2 and 5 centimeters (three-quarters of an inch to 2 inches). The cancer has not spread to the lymph nodes under the arm.

  o The tumor is between 2 and 5 centimeters (three-quarters of an inch to 2 inches). The cancer has spread to the lymph nodes under the arm.

  o The tumor is larger than 5 centimeters (2 inches). The cancer has not spread to the lymph nodes under the arm.

- **Stage III** is locally advanced cancer. It is divided into Stage IIIA, IIIB, and IIIC.

- **Stage IIIA** is one of the following:
  - The tumor is no more than 5 centimeters (2 inches) across. The cancer has spread to underarm lymph nodes that are attached to each other or to other structures. Or the cancer may have spread to lymph nodes behind the breastbone.
  - The tumor is more than 5 centimeters across. The cancer has spread to underarm lymph nodes that are either alone or attached to each other or to other structures. Or the cancer may have spread to lymph nodes behind the breastbone.
- **Stage IIIB** is a tumor of any size that has grown into the chest wall or the skin of the breast. It may be associated with swelling of the breast or with nodules (lumps) in the breast skin:
  - The cancer may have spread to lymph nodes under the arm.
  - The cancer may have spread to underarm lymph nodes that are attached to each other or other structures. Or the cancer may have spread to lymph nodes behind the breastbone.
  - Inflammatory breast cancer is a rare type of breast cancer. The breast looks red and swollen because cancer cells block the lymph vessels in the skin of the breast. When a doctor diagnoses inflammatory breast cancer, it is at least Stage IIIB, but it could be more advanced.
- **Stage IIIC** is a tumor of any size. It has spread in one of the following ways:
  - The cancer has spread to the lymph nodes behind the breastbone and under the arm.
  - The cancer has spread to the lymph nodes above or below the collarbone.

- **Stage IV** is distant metastatic cancer. The cancer has spread to other parts of the body, such as the bones or liver.

Recurrent cancer is cancer that has come back after a period of time when it could not be detected. Even when the cancer seems to be completely destroyed, the disease sometimes returns because undetected cancer cells remained somewhere in your body after treatment. It may return in the breast or chest wall. Or it may return in any other part of the body, such as the bones, liver, lungs, or brain.

About the Authors

In 1982, Aley Abraham became the first in her family to come to the U.S. Already an established tenth-grade teacher with two Indian bachelor degrees, she went back to school in the U.S. and earned a degree in medical technology. Today she works as a microbiologist at Children's Medical Center in Dallas, Texas. Aley is an active volunteer with The American Cancer Society and speaks frequently at her local church. She has been married for 39 years, has two daughters, two sons-in-law, and one granddaughter.

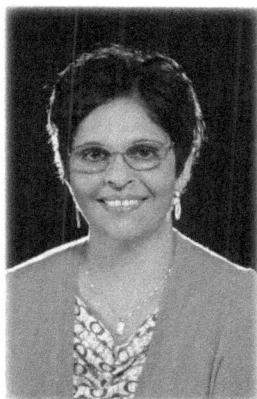

As an active wife, mother and career professional, Susan Abraham Thomas enjoys the opportunity to write. She has written for school newspapers and journals, company newsletters and online blogs; created original greeting cards; and supplies daily devotionals. Susan holds a Bachelor of Science degree in Computer Engineering from Texas A&M University and is a certified PMP.

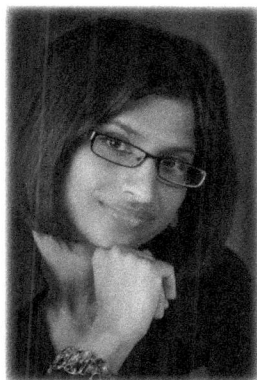

www.ingramcontent.com/pod-product-compliance
Lightning Source LLC
Chambersburg PA
CBHW031158270326
41931CB00006B/315